Delmar's LPN/LVN Review Series: *Mental Health*

Gary W. Stogsdill

Director of Staff Development
Assistant Director of Nursing Services
Laurel Ridge Hospital
San Antonio, Texas

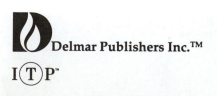

Delmar Publishers Inc.™

I(T)P™

Notice to the Reader

Delmar Staff
  Publisher: David Gordon
  Sponsoring Editor: Elisabeth F. Williams
  Project Editor: Carol Micheli
  Production Coordinator: Barbara A. Bullock
  Art/Design Coordinator: Mary Siener

For information, address Delmar Publishers Inc.
3 Columbia Circle, Box 15-015
Albany, New York 12212

Printed in the United States of America
Published simultaneously in Canada by Nelson Canada, a division of the Thomson Corporation

1 2 3 4 5 6 7 8 9 10 11 XXX 01 00 99 98 97 96 95

Library of Congress Cataloging-in-Publication Data
Stogsdill, Gary W.
    Delmar's LPN/LVN Review Series: Mental health / Gary W. Stogsdill. — 1st ed.
        p.   cm. — (Delmar's LPN/LVN review series)
    Includes index and disk.
    ISBN 0-8273-5698-6 (text and disk.)
    1. Psychiatric nursing.   I. Title.   II. Series
    [DNLM: 1. Mental Disorders—nursing. 2. Psychiatric Nursing—
methods.   WY 160 S873m 1995]
RC440.S786 1995
610.73'68—dc20
DNLM/DLC
for Library of Congress   93-43479
                                                                     CIP

CONTENTS

PREFACE

This textbook is written for:

• The graduate Practical/Vocational nurse to assist in the preparation for the State Boards;

• As a guide to the entry level Practical/Vocational Nurse in the clinical or employment setting;

• As a general introduction to Mental Health for other technical workers in the Mental Health field;

• Those who want to find out more about mental health.

This text is a comprehensive review of mental health knowledge for these practitioners. With the additional feature of having singular, measurable, and objective learning goals. This text also follows the APIE nursing process format. Briefly stated, the learner will be able to: (1) contribute to the assessment component of the nursing care plan by collecting subjective and objective data; (2) assist the Professional Nurse with the preparation of a plan of care; (3) assist with the implementation of nursing care; and (4) with assistance from the professional nurse, evaluate care of the outcome of the plan of care.

The text is written in the format that I have developed in teaching student nurses. For the graduate who is studying for the Practical Nurse/Vocational Nurse State Boards this book should prove to be an invaluable asset. Previous students have successfully passed the State Boards at a rate of 98% annually.

Each chapter is structured as follows:

    Contents of Chapter

    Key Chapter Objectives

    Definitions

    Competency list

At the end of each chapter you will find the following:

• A summary of key concepts. The focus is on the materials that could appear on the NCLEX-PN examination.

• At least 10 review questions. Chapter XI, Psychotropic Medications, has 101 medication questions. These questions **are not** from the NCLEX examination, but are similar in structure and content. There are 200 NCLEX-PN relevant questions.

Preparing for the computerized NCLEX

Start preparing for the NCLEX at the beginning of the second semester or after the first block of course work at the beginning of the medical surgical course, whichever occurs first. Review this book and lecture notes each evening for at least two hours. Each evening includes seven days a week, weekends, holidays, and breaks in the education program. Warning!! If you wait until the semester before graduating, you will have handicapped your preparation.

Admission to the NCLEX

You will submit an Application for Licensure to the Board of Nursing for approval for Licensure. After the application is approved by the Board of Nursing, you will receive an Authorization to Test. You will then call the center of your choice and schedule a testing date and time, which may be Monday through Saturday (and Sundays if necessary). If you are taking the NCLEX for the first time, you will be scheduled within 30 days (if you choose) of your call to the testing center. If you are repeating the examination, you will be scheduled within 45 days of your call. Testing is available 15 hours a day and 6 (or in some cases, 7 days) a week. Testing is to be done at Sylvan Technology Centers. There should be no more than 10 persons testing at the same time.

Listen carefully to the directions given by the test proctors at the time of the NCLEX. The NCLEX-PN is now administered using computerized adaptive testing known as CAT. This means that the multiple choice questions are assembled interactively as the test progresses. As the test progresses, a competency score accumulates based on answers to previous questions. The testing continues until a pass or fail score can definitely be determined mathematically. At that point the test stops. You will be notified of the pass or fail in a matter of weeks.

At the testing center, you will receive instructions as to how to apply to take the NCLEX—from your nursing program, your state licensing entity, and directly from the testing center representatives. You be required to schedule yourself directly with the testing center within 30 days of notification of eligibility for the NCLEX.

There is no requirement for you to be computer literate. You will need to use two keys on the computer keyboard—the enter/return key and the space bar. The enter key is used to accept the answer you have selected and the space bar is used to move from answer to answer. Once you have pressed the enter/return key, you will be asked if you are sure that this is the answer you have selected. If you answer by depressing the enter key one more time, that will be the answer you select. If you decide you don't want that selection, then when the question is asked, "is this the answer you choose?" you would press the space bar and begin the process of selecting the correct answer. Prior to the NCLEX-PN you will be provided with a tutorial and actual hands-on experience. The tutorial will be the total learning you need to take the NCLEX.

1. You will have a maximum of 5 hours (300 minutes) to answer as many of the 180 "real" questions (questions that are a part of your score) and 25 "tryouts" (questions that are being tested for inclusion in later NCLEX examinations) as you can. The maximum number of questions that any one candidate will have to answer is 205. You should be answering questions at a rate of one question every 1 1/2 minutes. *Once you have answered a question and the computer has accepted it, you cannot return to that question for any reason.* As you are taking the test, the computer program is calculating scores on the basis of your answers. Your test may end at one of the following three points: a. when the computer program computes that it is mathematically impossible for you to pass the examination, b. when the program computes that you have achieved competency by correctly answering the required questions, or c. when the test time has expired. Practice your tests and examinations at a rate of 1 question every 1 1/2 minutes (90 seconds).

2. All of the NCLEX examination questions are in multiple choice format. There are no matching, fill in the blanks, etc.—only multiple choice. In fact, there are no answer sheets. Practice answering multiple choice questions.

3. Be consistent with your review when preparing for the NCLEX. Start your NCLEX preparation when you start your Medical-Surgical block at the beginning of the second unit of your program. If you will set aside no more than 2 hours a day for review, for at least 6 months *before* you take the NCLEX, you should have ample time to prepare. The NCLEX is given monthly at testing centers located throughout the United States. Your review for the NCLEX should begin as early in your program as possible, but at least 6 months prior to graduation. Should you not successfully complete the NCLEX, you should double your time frame for review from 2 to 4 hours per day. Prepare for the NCLEX *before* not *after* you have taken it.

4. Answer all the NCLEX questions with your best effort. You will be given the opportunity to change your answer one time, and then it's on to the next question. If absolutely nothing comes to your mind, guess if you have to. Once the computer has accepted your answer, you may not change it. a. For NCLEX purposes, references to the Registered Nurse in this book refer to the relationship between the practical/vocational nurse after graduation. Please think of yourself as a Licensed Practical or Licensed Vocational Nurse and remember you are no longer a student. b. The NCLEX uses the term Registered Nurse as a legal (by state law) relation to the Practical/Vocational nurse. The term Registered Nurse on the NCLEX does not refer to your faculty.

General hints for all multiple choice tests

1. Read each question carefully. There will be no multiple-multiple or negatively phrased questions. Each question is free standing and does not conform to the situation-style format used in the recent past.

2. Look for key words in the question such as except, primary, initial, least, or first.

3. While you are reading the question, begin to formulate a possible answer.

4. With your possible answer in mind, quickly review the answers in the test to see if any of them match.

5. If your answer is a match, enter the answer, and at the computer prompt, accept it. The computer will then present you with the next question.

6. If your answer is not among the answers given, read the question again.

7. Eliminate the obviously incorrect answers.

8. From the remaining answers, choose the closest match.

9. Don't become discouraged or anxious. It may seem that the first few questions don't have a correct answer. That's just anxiety, and is fairly common among test takers. Those questions do have a correct answer. You will be able to respond after you have become accustomed to the computer environment.

10. The NCLEX is a composite of questions from several different test writers who use several different textbooks. There may be questions that you have never heard before you take the examination. The more you review, the more

likely it is you will be able to answer most or all of the questions.

11. It is better to guess and answer the question than to leave a question unanswered.

12. Remember, the answer you select must be therapeutic and safe.

13. Try to pace yourself so that you do not let too much time elapse for each question.

14. Be certain that the answer you select is the one that agrees with the question.

15. When you have selected your answer, *you can not change it.*

16. You should be able to eliminate two of the four choices of answers for each question.

Acknowledgments

I would like to express my sincerest thanks to all those who assisted me in the preparation of this work.

Marion Waldman, my editor.

Leona J. Knight, RN, MS, a valued colleague who never failed to review any of the content.

Jane Stillabower, RN, MSN who, even though she was recovering from major surgery, certainly made my thoughts more clear.

Virgina Rye, RN, MSN, who shared her years of psychiatric experiences, both teaching and clinical with me and reviewed materials unceasingly.

Sandra Avenell-Brown, RN, MSN who helped lead me through the content as it was being developed.

Dr. George Nicolaou MD, Board Certified Psychiatrist, who frequently gave me reality therapy.

A special thanks to Patricia Lyons RN, MSN, who reviewed the content and actually enjoyed doing it.

To the Alamo Community College District for the precious "educational endeavor" time it so generously allowed. Without the assistance of the district this work would not have been possible.

Reviewers

Kathy Neeb, RN
LPN Nursing Instructor
Minneapolis Tech College

Karen B. Robinson, RN, MA
ADN/VN Instructor
Temple Junior College

Yvonne B. Meinket
Program Supervisor—Health Occupations
Charlotte Vocational Technical Center

Bernice Rudolph, BS, RN, PHN
Senior Instructor/Vocational Nursing
Casa Loma College

Mrs. JoAnn Dever, RN, MSN Ed
Chairperson PN Program
Indiana Vocational Technical College

INTRODUCTION

In the last 10 years of teaching Practical/Vocational students, I have collected a diversity of teaching lecture materials. In 1988, I observed that the students State Board pass rate was fairly consistently 100%. Both students and faculty prevailed on me to tell them how I achieved such high State Board results. I discovered that the materials I taught from contained certain critical materials that one way or another always appeared on the State Boards. Although the basics have sometimes been altered, the basics are still identified in A, P, I, and E. These letters represent Assess, Plan, Implement, and Evaluate, which is the nursing process for LPN/LVN. As you proceed through this text keep these elements in mind. Although this text is all about mental health, the APIE works in any course.

The underlying theme, comes from my lecture notes when I was a student nurse. I was fortunate to have been taught Psychiatric Nursing by Elizabeth Helm, RN, Kansas City Psychiatric Receiving Center, which was one component of the Kansas City General Hospital and Medical Center, in Kansas City, Missouri, February, March and April, 1963.

Dedication

This book is dedicated to my parents
Joseph E. Stogsdill 1908-1968
Vivian E. Stogsdill 1908-1964

and to my sister
Karen Gayle Stogsdill Heston, RN
a truly great sister and a resourceful colleague.

CHAPTER 1

Foundations of Mental Health

KEY CHAPTER OBJECTIVES

Upon completion of Chapter 1, the student should be able to:

- Identify characteristics (key features) of the mentally healthy and the mentally ill.
- Identify the evolution of mental health.
- Identify milestones in mental health.
- Identify the key components of the community health movement.
- Identify the various components of personality during development.
- Identify factors that may influence the developing personality.
- Personality Development
   Freud
   Erickson
- Identify defense mechanisms.
   Define defense mechanisms.
   Identify the purposes of defense mechanisms.
- Identify responses to stressors of life.
- Identify emotional responses to stress, illness and other life events.
- Identify sexual disorders.
- Identify the sexual response cycle.

DEFINITIONS

HEALTH: The absence of disease, physiologic, psychologic, genetic, or acquired from the environment.

MENTAL HEALTH: Mental health is "psychologic well being or adequate adjustment, particularly as such adjustment conforms to the community accepted standards of human relations."[1] Specific characteristics of the mentally healthy person are discussed later in this chapter.

MENTAL ILLNESS: The lack or absence of the ability to adjust or adapt behavior that is or would be acceptable to community standards of human relations. Alteration from the acceptable standards of behavior.

EVOLUTION OF THE MENTAL HEALTH DELIVERY SYSTEM

A. Mental illness is a major health problem in the United States. One-third of all individuals experience some form of mental illness during a period of their life. The most common mental illness is depression.

B. There has been an ever-increasing number of patients admitted to mental hospitals or special units in private hospitals.

C. Mental illness might be said to be the extent to which problems are not dealt with through rational decisions.

D. A system of standards has been developed for assessment of patient care in the mental health system. These may be found in the State Department of Health (Human Resources) or in the mental health codes of your state.

Attributes of mentally healthy persons are that they:

A. Solve problems

B. Have self direction

C. Have a feeling of well-being

D. Are productive

E. Enjoy all aspects of life

F. Set goals and limits for activities

G. Accept and express love

H. Are able to cope with crisis without help from other than family and friends

I. Respect self and others

J. Are flexible, adaptable, and willing to try new things.

---

[1] Campbell, Robert J. *Psychiatric Dictionary*, 5th ed., Oxford University Press, New York, 1981.

Attributes of mentally ill persons are that they:

A. Have unstable mental processes

B. Exhibit illness by behavioral dysfunction

C. Become more and more limited in their social interaction

D. Have eventual disorganization of self (thoughts) as evidenced by unusual or significant changes in behavior. Examples of causes of behavioral changes that may indicate pending mental illness:

   1. Threatened by specific object or person

   2. Disrupting of relationship(s)

   3. Abnormal suspiciousness

   4. Heightened fear(s)

   5. Increased anger or rage—with or without outbursts

   6. General unhappiness with or withdrawal from the milieu. *The milieu is defined as a therapeutic environment conducive to psychological treatment to restore appropriate social behaviors (functioning).*

HISTORIC PERSPECTIVES OF MENTAL HEALTH THROUGHOUT THE AGES

A. Primitive times

   1. Those who did not conform to the norm were possessed by evil spirits that had to be driven out.

   2. Combinations of treatments were used, all treatments were administered by medicine men (witches—warlocks).

B. Ancient Greeks, Romans, and Arabs

   1. Viewed mental illness as a natural occurrence

   2. Treated mentally ill humanely

   3. Plato, 400 B.C., a Greek, believed that family should care for the mentally ill.

   4. Hippocrates, 460 B.C., a Greek, believed that all disease had bodily causes and that mental illness was caused by excessive bile.

C. Middle ages

   1. Reverted back to witchcraft and superstition.

   2. Mentally ill were usually locked in asylums and starved and tortured; blood letting was done to release the evil spirits.

D. The Renaissance

   1. Evil spirits possessed the body.

   2. The mentally ill were considered harmful to society and they were imprisoned.

   3. Mental illness was considered irreversible.

4. Punitive measures, such as physical beatings or isolation in cages or closets, were used for behavioral changes.

5. All rights were forfeited.

6. First hospital for the mentally ill was established in England in the 1600s.

   a. Patients were kept chained in cages.

   b. For a small fee, the public could view the patients.

   c. The nickname "bedlam" was derived from St. Mary's of Bethlehem Hospital.

E. The 1700s

1. In France, the chains were removed but patients were still confined within institutions.

2. In colonial America, the mentally ill were publicly humiliated by whipping and dunking. Others were burned at the stake as they were considered to be witches, or possessed by the devil or demons.

F. The 1800s

1. Mentally ill were treated more humanely.

2. Discoveries that certain vitamin deficiencies and some diseases could contribute to mental illness, for example, high fever can induce a state of delirium.

G. The 1900s

1. Early beginnings of the mental health movement.

2. Various states began building hospitals for the mentally ill.

3. The introduction of short-term care.

4. An emphasis was placed on prevention of mental illness.

5. Eventually the development of the goal to return the patient to society was identified and implemented.

Important Milestones in the Care of the Mentally Ill

A. Theories related to mental processes began to evolve.

1. Sigmund Freud, M.D. (1856–1939), Vienna, Austria, founded the principles of psychoanalysis based on id, ego, and superego arising from "Psychosexual Development." The underlying mental illness was the result of sexual imbalance, either excess or inadequacy that occurred during the developmental process.

2. H.S. Sullivan (1892–1949), United States, founded the School of Interpersonal Psychiatry based on the theory that personality is the result of interpersonal relationships or psychosocial development.

3. E. H. Erickson (1902–   ), a social psychoanalyst from the United States, developed a "Cultural" theory based on the application of psychoanalytic techniques to social and anthropological (human) studies.

4. J. Piaget (1896–1980), France, a developmental psychologist who arrived at an "Intellectual" theory.

5. B. F. Skinner (1904–1990), United States, started the "Behavioral" theory.

B. Important contributors to the advancement of mental health

1. Benjamin Rush, M.D. (1746–1813), Pennsylvania, "Father of American Psychiatry," stressed human treatment and the importance of occupational therapy.

2. Philippe Pinel, M.D. (1745–1826), France, advocated the removal of chains and pressed for humane treatment of the mentally ill.

3. William Tuke, philanthropist (1732–1822), began the reform movement by providing money and establishing an institution for humane treatment of the mentally ill in York, England.

4. Dorothea Lynde Dix, school teacher and social reformer (1802–1887). An American from the New England area. Through lobbying, she was able to promote the care of the mental health patient and get legislative passage of laws that established state hospitals, secured the release of prisoners to the mental health facilities, and generally promoted the appropriate treatment of the mentally ill.

5. Charles Dickens, author (1812–1870), England, wrote about social injustice and social needs in England and America, and greatly influenced reformers of the time.

6. Clifford Beers, humanitarian (1876–1943), author of *A Mind That Found Itself*. The book was written to provide a description of the patients' perspectives of the effects of being confined to a mental hospital, and urged for better treatment of mentally ill patients during inpatient treatment. Later Beers became a founding voice of the National Society for Mental Hygiene; which evolved into the National Association for Mental Health.

7. The National Mental Health Act of 1946 provided for the National Institute of Mental Health in 1948. It expanded the existing mental health care delivery system and provided financial resources to increase research and education directed at improving treatment and rehabilitation of mental health patients.

8. The 1963 Mental Retardation Facilities and Community Mental Health Center Construction Act provided federal matching funds to states to build community health centers.

9. Currently, several settings are available for those requiring mental health care.

   a. Long-term care (more than 30 days)

   b. Acute care (generally less than 30 days)

   c. Psychiatric intensive care unit (PICU)

    d. Psychiatric units within a general hospital setting

    e. Partial (day) treatment programs

    f. Crisis intervention centers

    g. Halfway houses

    h. Counseling centers

    i. 1-800 hot lines

    j. Residential treatment centers

    k. community mental health centers.

COMMUNITY MENTAL HEALTH MOVEMENT

A. The National Mental Health Act placed emphasis on the quality of care received by hospitalized mentally ill patients.

B. It also emphasized the level of skills necessary to deliver higher quality care and lower the rate of hospitalizing chronically ill patients.

C. The objective of the Act was to alter the state hospital model that linked chronicity and severity of mental disease to the length of hospitalization. (Some chronically mentally ill patients lived most of their lives in state mental hospitals.)

D. Primary objectives of the Community Mental Act are to prevent mental illness, cope with symptoms of illness, and return the patient to the community as soon as possible.

DEVELOPMENT OF THE PERSONALITY

The mind or psyche operates in three distinct areas or territories, conscious, subconscious, and unconscious, which are parts of the underlying personality. These three areas contain the total of the person's personality.

A. *Conscious*: holds all past experiences in a state of easy recall. Those experiences are easily recalled and pose minimal emotional discomfort.

B. *Subconscious*: these are unpleasant feelings that are deliberately pushed out of the conscious level. These feelings can be recalled, but only with considerable effort. These thoughts may cause some uneasy feelings depending on the underlying cause or event that leads to the feelings and/or thoughts.

C. *Unconscious*: the storehouse of unwanted thoughts and feelings.

    1. These thoughts cannot be brought back to the conscious level at will, they are too unacceptable to be permitted return to the conscious level.

    2. If these thoughts and feelings are returned to the conscious level, they will cause or have the potential to cause severe anxiety.

3. The longer these feelings and thoughts are suppressed in the unconscious, the more difficult it will be to release them into the conscious.

D. Maslow identified a hierarchy of needs: from lowest to highest levels of needs

1. Physiologic (survival) needs such as food, water, sex, shelter

2. Safety and security needs such as protecting oneself against harm or deprivation

3. Affection and social needs such as association with, companionship or fulfilling the need to belong, for example, groups, friendships

4. Esteem needs such as awareness of the need for self-respect, acceptance, and knowing that one has importance relating to others

5. Actualization needs such as fulfillment of one's potential. Humans seek to be creative and to be able to express themselves uniquely. Self-actualization is the highest level of Maslow's hierarchy.

THEORIES RELATED TO PERSONALITY

DEFINITIONS

ID: (Freudian) That part of the personality structure that contains unconscious and instinctual drives, urges, and desires. The instant gratification that only operates in the "me" mode

EGO: (Freudian) That part of the personality structure that is the sum of mental processes such as perception and memory. The ego is the mediator between the id and the superego. The ego is the self. The area of the personality where conflicts are resolved by compromise between the powerful forces of the id and the superego. The ego is reality oriented.

SUPEREGO: (Freudian) That part of the personality that contains ethical, moral standards, and self-criticism judgments and values. When values and standards are applied to childhood dreams and wishes, the conscious begins to emerge.

PERSONALITY: Consistent attitudes and behaviors. The ability to adapt to the environment and derive satisfaction from that relationship. Finally, it is the ingraining of patterns of behavior that evolves consciously and unconsciously from life experiences and includes strengths (assets) and weaknesses (liabilities).

Factors That Influence the Developing Personality

A. Genetic factors

B. Interactions with the environment

C. Nurturing

1. Early emotional experiences

2. Relations/interactions with parents

D. Order of birth; oldest to youngest, or only child

E. Identification with parent(s) by adopting parents' attitudes, standards, behaviors, values, and philosophies. The incorporation of behavioral characteristics, both consciously and unconsciously, that are learned by interactions with parent(s). For example, if a child sees that her/his parents are not working for whatever reason, then he/she may presume that this is acceptable adult behavior.

F. Encountering emotional problems involving security, love, aggression, dependence, or rebellion against authority.

G. Life experiences will ultimately foster personality growth or block/distort the healthy personality

Importance of Personality Development to the Nurse

A. During periods of stress, physical illness, or mental illness the patient is likely to regress (see Defense Mechanisms).

B. Early recognition of deviations from normal behavior can lead to early intervention. For instance—

1. When a normally very independent person becomes very dependent and demanding

2. When the child, who is completely toilet trained, suddenly regresses to infant elimination; this may be an overt sign of threat or stress. This can happen, for example, when a new child or baby is brought into the home.

C. You should be aware of how your personality was formed.

The Stages of Personality Development According to Freud

See definitions of id, ego, and superego.

A. Id

1. Part of the personality controlled by the pleasure principle.

2. Consists of the body's primitive, uncivilized, and basic biological drives and instincts and is concerned *only* with achieving and maintaining a state of satisfaction and pleasure. The immediate gratification is a part of the id. These gratifications may be physical, emotional, or a combination.

3. Is subconscious and unconscious and is necessary for survival.

4. Newborns are little bundles of id.

B. Ego

1. Is the component of the psyche that operates in reality. Psyche is the mind, not to be confused with the brain, the physical structure.

2. "Self" or conscious awareness.

3. Satisfaction is achieved in a manner that coincides with physical and social reality.

4. Defers immediate gratification for delayed satisfactions.

5. The ego mediates or arbitrates struggles between the id and the superego. There is a constant struggle between "good" and "evil" as to which will dominate the ultimate behavior of the individual.

6. At about 6 months the "I" and "me" (id) begins to evolve into the ego. This is the beginning of the "we" or ego phase of personality development.

C. Superego

1. Conscious

2. Judgmental

3. Hyper self-critical, hypermoral, and self-punishing

4. Reinforced by teachers, clergy, and learned from parents via role modeling

5. Violation of superego may cause guilt varying from mild to severe

D. If conflict between id and superego cannot be resolved, anxiety is the primary result. This intrapsychic conflict is mediated (balanced) by the ego. If there are continuous unresolved conflicts, these conflicts may eventually lead to some degree of breakdown in interpersonal relationships and/or personality.

E. Stages of personality development (Freud)

1. Oral stage (birth to 1 year)

   a. Id function

   b. The mouth and lips are the erogenous zones; sucking, taking objects into the mouth. The definition of erogenous is pleasure giving, based on pleasure seeking. The pleasure derived from stimulation of the erogenous zone(s) is emotional or physical gratification.

2. Anal stage (1–2 years)

   a. The anal/genital areas are the erogenous zones

   b. Ambivalence; I love you, I hate you

   c. Elimination gives pleasure

   d. Beginning of magical thinking (probably to relieve anxiety or escape from stressors) and/or temper tantrums when not satisfied or not gratified. This may also be the beginning of attempts to control the surroundings by controlling bowel elimination (an attention-seeking technique).

3. Oedipal stage (3–5 years)

   a. Each child goes through a stage of strong attraction to the parent of the opposite sex, accompanied by jealousy of the parent of the same sex. The Oedipus complex is briefly discussed here.

1) A boy has strong feelings for his mother and simultaneously has feelings of jealousy, hate, and fear of his father. If the mother were to become sexually aroused by her son's stimulation, then the son becomes the lover, and the mother becomes extremely overprotective of her son. The son wishes for the father to go away or die.

2) The opposite of the oedipal complex: daughters have strong feelings for the father and negative feelings toward the mother—the Electra complex.

Note: Both the Oedipus and Electra complex were first described in the Greek play by Sophocles in Oedipus The King (495–406 B.C.).

b. If the situation is not managed with understanding by the parents, the result may be a permanent attachment for the parent of the opposite sex. If the father becomes sexually aroused by the daughter, incest, rape, or other forms of molestation could result.

c. Superego develops.

4. Latency period (6–12 years)

a. Quiet personality growth

b. Child identifies more the with parent of the same sex

c. Balance between freedom and control

5. Genital stage (12–18 years)

a. Daydreaming and wishful thinking emerge about sexual encounters and how to manage these imagined encounters

b. Hero worship

c. Formation of heterosexual versus homosexual roles, which later may become the acceptable sex identity. Recent studies indicate that homosexual traits may be linked to genetics. Previously, most authorities speculated that homosexual behaviors were environmentally influenced.

The Stages of Personality Development According to Erickson

Note: Very few of us develop in accordance with a fixed schedule of events. We are individuals and tend to develop at our own distinct rates. Although rates may vary, we do tend to pass through each of these described phases, but at our own rate.

A. Infancy—Period of Trust (birth to 18 months)

1. Primary needs are acquiring a sense of basic trust while overcoming a sense of basic mistrust.

2. Emotional environment is evaluated through the satisfaction of oral needs and through physical contact.

B. Toddler—Period of autonomy (18 months to 3 or 4 years)

1. Concept of being worthy of love is of primary importance.

2. Primary significant person is the mother unless she is not present. If the mother is not present, then an alternate significant person fills the mother role.

3. Needs to be met are:

   a. Biological

      1) Food

      2) Shelter

      3) Warmth

   b. Psychological

      1) Security

      2) Acceptance

      3) Love

4. If needs are met, the infant learns to trust and tolerate occasional frustrations of delays in gratification.

5. If needs are not met, the results may be feelings of being unloved and not accepted. The child will become distrustful, unloving, and nonaccepting.

   a. The child becomes demanding, fearful, hostile, cold, and withdrawn.

   b. Schizophrenics share feelings of being unloved and unwanted in the early stages of development.

C. Toddler stage (18 months to 3 years)

1. Autonomy is the primary developmental focus.

2. Adapts to social and moral norms.

   a. Completes bowel and bladder training.

   b. Begins to distinguish sexual differences of parents. May imitate parent of same sex.

3. Interacts with parents to begin to establish and test personality boundaries. What can and cannot be gotten away with?

   a. If interaction is constructive, outcome will be independence.

   b. If deprived of learning experiences, it is possible the child will develop a sense of shame, doubt, and expect defeat. This deprivation is not a onetime event, but rather a continual process or series of deprivations. Continual deprivation may result in some degree of dependence, hence, a codependent personality type.

D. Preschool (3–5 years)

1. A major stressor of preschoolers is development of role identity.
   a. Imagination is used freely to resolve stress and conflict.
   b. Play is the work of children; play is important.
   c. Curiosity; fantasy leads to normal development, however, if the initiative is blocked for whatever reason, guilt, or shame may be the result.

2. Independence and dependence are ambivalent feelings at this age.

D. Later childhood (6–11 years)
   1. The major stress is the emerging socialization role.
      a. Wants to participate in creative activities with others.
      b. Accepts instruction and needs recognition to enjoy work.
      c. Inferiority may develop if attention and recognition are insufficient.
   2. Must learn to interact with peers.
   3. Acceptance by peer group is important.
   4. Period of transition from child to adolescence.

E. Adolescence (12–18 years)
   1. Self-identification and sexual development are the primary stressors.
      a. Experiences rapid body growth and physical development.
      b. Emotions and sexual feelings (urges) become heightened. Curious about the obvious anatomic changes that are in progress. Anxious about when the changes will stop. Begins to seek sex information from peers or parents — any source that is available.
   2. Period of ambivalence
      a. Seeks independence from family controls, yet still needs security.
      b. Has considerable self-doubt of own ability; at other times, is absolutely certain of own abilities.
      c. Begins to feel pressure for identifying occupation, but says "I will just be a beach bum" or "I don't know."
      d. Begins to install own standards and values in opposition to parents wishes.
      e. Identifies with and finds security in peer group, such as gangs or those who share similar views, for example, those who love rock and roll music or those who are trying to gain independence from parents.
   3. This is a critical time in terms of interactions of the adolescent and the parent; communication that reflects trust and concern is of utmost importance.
   4. All components of environment, biologic self, socialization, culture, and all other components become unified. If this does not occur then the result may be an alteration in the mental processes ranging from slight to severe—defiance, dissociation, or indifference are possibilities

F. Adulthood (early 19–24 years)
   1. Intimacy in relationships predominates.

  2. Accepts and gives love (emotional).

  3. Commitment and marriage formalize relationship.

G. Middle adulthood (25 – 65 years)

  1. Involved in and committed to career and child rearing.

  2. Begins to look forward to the future generation.

  3. Isolation may result if an intimate relationship is not developed.

H. Late adulthood (65+ years)

  1. Time of fulfillment, retrospective vision acute.

  2. Enjoyment of earned benefits.

  3. If there has been no intimate relationship or the person has not accepted previous wins or losses, then it is likely that there will be some degree of regret, despair, loneliness, or helplessness.

DEFENSE MECHANISMS

DEFINITION

DEFENSE MECHANISMS, OR ADJUSTMENT TECHNIQUES: Methods that are used by an individual to relieve or decrease anxieties produced by an uncomfortable situation that threatens self or psyche. Defense mechanisms are used to resolve intrapsychic conflicts and thereby relieve stress. Defense mechanisms are psychological short-cuts for preservation of self. Some defense mechanisms are constructive, whereas others are more destructive in terms of the eventual behavioral outcome.

Using Defense Mechanisms

A. The purpose of defense mechanisms (adjustment techniques) is to continually attempt to reduce anxiety and reestablish psychological equilibrium.

B. An individual's adjustment depends on the ability to vary responses so that he/she can deal with anxiety.

C. Individuals use essentially the same defense techniques. Although the exact use may vary from individual to individual to resolve intrapsychic conflicts, the mechanisms are fundamentally the same. Mentally healthy individuals tend to use the defense mechanisms in a positive way. Mentally unhealthy persons tend to use defense mechanisms in a less than socially acceptable way or for a self-serving purpose.

D. The exercise of a defense mechanism may be a conscious process, but it is usually generated at the unconscious level.

E. Adjustment techniques are compromise solutions that include many different forms and offer alternative solutions to problems.

F. Healthy adjustment mechanisms may include rationalization, sublimation, compensation, and suppression. (See definitions that follow.)

   1. A healthy adjustment is characterized by:

      a. The infrequent need to use unconscious adjustment techniques.

      b. The ability to form new responses necessary to meet new problems.

      c. The ability to change the external environment.

      d. The ability to modify one's own needs.

   2. Defense mechanisms are partially environmental and partially genetic. No one has an exact number to attach to which part is environmental and which part is genetic.

G. Unhealthy adjustment to life events

   1. An unhealthy adjustment is characterized by:

      a. The inability or loss of ability to initiate or to initiate or vary responses.

      b. The individual's retreat from the problem or from reality.

      c. Continual use of unhealthy defense mechanisms that may eventually interfere with maintenance of self-image.

   2. Unhealthy adjustment mechanisms may include regression, repression, denial, projection, and isolation.

   3. Mentally ill persons use defense mechanisms to avoid problems rather than solving them, sometimes resulting in inappropriate behavior.

   4. Defense mechanisms are used to maintain balance between the person and her/his relationship to the environment and with others.

H. Defense mechanisms are used by most people in one form or another.

The 20 Most Common Defense Mechanisms

A. Compensation: Used to cover up an area of weakness by showing a great deal of strength or excellence in another area.

Example: A high school student is physically weak and considers her/himself ugly, constantly studies and becomes the valedictorian of her/his class.

B. Conversion: Strong emotional (intrapsychic) conflicts become physical symptoms (motor or sensory, or both)

Example: A student who is not prepared for a final examination develops a severe headache on the day of the examination.

C. Denial (negation): Refusal to face reality or the rejection of obvious facts or truth, operates best in a weak ego system. Probably the most commonly used of all defense mechanisms.

Example: Refusal to see a physician because the patient does not want to know the truth about an apparent problem.

D. Displacement: Transfer of internalized feelings from the object of origin or conflict to an object that poses no threat.

Example: Your superior at work yells at you, when you get home you yell at your significant other or kick the dog.

E. Dissociation: Detachment or splitting certain thoughts or processes from the psyche in an attempt to stabilize psychic interactions. Dissociation may include a loss, either temporary or permanent, depending on the ability to rejoin the separated psyche. May result in multiple personalities depending on the depth of the splitting and independence of the "split" part.

Example: The patient observes that rather than becoming a part of the situation, such as not allowing oneself to become involved in a serious and meaningful relationship due to a previous very painful relationship and fear of being hurt again, leads to superficial behavior(s) and shallow relationships. One component of the patients identity has been severed and is being dealt with in another completely separate and different part of the mind.

F. Fantasy: Gratification by wishful thinking, daydreaming, imagined sequential events or mental images, serves to resolve unconscious conflicts.

Example: If you do that, I'll do _____, or "I should have said."

G. Fixation: One component of psychosocial development is delayed or nullified, behavioral development ceases because of lack of or an excess of gratification.

Example: A 10-year-old sucks her/his thumb while taking an exam or an adult behaves like a high school student, failing to move beyond that period of time when, as an athlete, the patient was very popular and very satisfied with her/himself.

H. Identification: An unconscious internalization of another's desirable personality attributes or traits.

Example: Admiration of a religious person causes a person to be pious—a desirable quality—strengthens superego, or a teenager's need to belong to the peer group causes her/him to adopt the group behavior (hair style, clothes, footwear).

I. Insulation: Passive withdrawal. Prevents further intrusion by the offending person or object; selective environmental or emotional exclusion (may include relationships).

Example: One, whose perception is that a relationship has ended in a disaster, will not quickly enter into another relationship; does not want to get hurt again, avoidance assures protection from the underlying cause of emotional conflict.

J. Introjection: Unconscious mechanism where love or hate objects symbolically become oneself.

Example: A depressed person believes that he/she is to blame for the evils of the world and to end the wickedness attempts suicide, unconsciously directing unacceptable hatred or aggression toward self, or a person reacts to the death of a loved one, not with anger, but with overwhelming grief or despair, resulting in underlying frustration.

K. Isolation: Unconscious separation of unacceptable impulse, idea, or act from its original memory source that reduces the original emotional charge.

Example: A person recalls that a terrible car accident occurred but has no recollection that a parent has died in the wreck.

L. Projection: Unconscious unacceptable emotions in the self are rejected and attributed or projected onto others.

Example: A child who has been spanked by the parent says "you hate me," or a student who fails a course states "I failed it because the teacher did not like me." This is an attempt to explain away the student's lack of study in that subject.

M. Rationalization: Unconscious operation whereby one attempts to justify conscious feelings, behaviors, or motives that would have been otherwise intolerable.

Example: "Oh well, it wasn't worth it anyway"—the sour grapes approach. An attempt to make our behavior more acceptable to ourselves and others.

N. Reaction formation: Unconscious mechanism in which a person takes on the attributes, i.e., affect, ideas, attitudes, and behaviors, that are the opposite of impulses or the underlying feelings.

Example: Excessive moral zeal may be a reaction to very strong but repressed asocial impulsiveness or a "good religious person" is also the town gossip.

O. Regression: Partial or symbolic return to a previous more comfortable time or feeling. A response (reaction) to a current stress or frustration. May be manifested in a number of ways including but not limited to bowel activity, thumb sucking, need for diapers, etc.

Example: A small child (6 years old who has long since completed bowel training) brings his mother a diaper, while sucking the thumb. When threatened, an adult may break into tears.

P. Repression: The unconscious process in which undesirable and unacceptable thoughts are kept from entering the conscious. The superego is the overriding psychic pressure.

Example: A child who is continually put down by overbearing parents, when grown, may be rebellious against any kind of authority. The individual may not be able to remember the name of a person about whom he/she has very strong negative feelings. Such feelings may include hate or guilt.

Q. Sublimation: Unconscious process whereby instinctual drives that are consciously unacceptable are diverted into personally and socially acceptable (constructive) channels.

Example: Artists sometime express very sexually explicit material on canvas and the art may be regarded as a masterpiece. A nurse who experiences extreme frustration in work relationships develops the strong need to play baseball or bowling at every opportunity to relieve the pent up hostility and/or frustrations.

R. Suppression: Consciously keeping unpleasant or unacceptable feelings, thoughts, impulses, or acts concealed. May result in frustration and/or guilt.

Example: Thinking that you want to do something unacceptable but consciously con-

cealing the thought; superego override of the thought or impulse. Deliberate attempt to push the unpleasant feelings out of the psyche. This is a conscious effort!

S. Symbolization: A general mechanism in all human thinking by which some mental representation comes to stand for some other thing, class of things, or attributes of something. This mechanism underlies dream formation and other similar symptoms, such as conversion reaction, obsessions, and compulsions. The link between the latent (underlying) meaning of the symptom and the symbol is usually unconscious.

Example: The cross is the symbol of Christianity. A wedding ring is the symbol of marriage. But both of these symbols have deeper underlying feelings or emotions strongly connected or linked to the symbol.

T. Undoing; Unconscious mechanism in which something unacceptable and already done is symbolically acted out in reverse, usually repetitiously, in the hope of relieving anxiety by reversing the first effect. The reverse of the process that caused the original unacceptable thought or act.

Example: Committing a murder and then becoming the person who is officially recognized as saving lives to undo the previous wrong.

Other commonly used defense mechanisms are compensation, confabulation, restitution, and substitution.

Nursing Care Associated With the Use of the Defense Mechanisms

A. Be aware of your own behavior and the use of adaptive techniques.

B. *Do not* criticize the patient's behavior and use of adjustive techniques. Modification of existing defense mechanisms may prove more beneficial than outright rejection of existing ones.

C. Assist the patient in learning new or alternative adjustive techniques for healthier adaptation.

D. Use techniques to help alleviate the patient's anxiety.

E. Do not attempt to arbitrarily eliminate adjustive techniques without replacement of healthier ones; they serve a purpose for the patient.

Remember *always; be nonthreatening, nonjudgmental, and no put-down.*

ASSESSING FOR STRESS

From the time we are conceived until the time we die, we all experience stress. It is with all of us each and every day. It assumes many forms, each form with a certain degree of mental involvement and response. The degree of involvement ranges from very mild stress to intolerable levels of stress. At times stress may even result in physical pain or somatic symptoms.

A. Sources of primary stress arising from events and experiences are:

    1. Developmental: Growing up; from neonate to adult has built-in stressors.

    2. Situational: During our lives we experience stress due to our environment, for example, flat tires in the middle of a 1000-mile trip.

B. The primary causes of stress are:

    1. Change

    2. Conflict

    3. Uncertainty

    4. Fear of failing

    5. Inability to control

    6. Unable to define purpose

    7. Some everyday stressors are:

        a. Hassles such as:

            1) Bad news

            2) Competition

            3) Deadlines

        b. Built-in stress (emotions) such as:

            1) Frustration(s)

            2) Guilt

            3) Perfectionism

        c. Overriding stressors that are built into life itself.

            1) Death and the accompanying grief

            2) Marital conflicts

            3) Interpersonal conflicts

            4) Financial concerns

        d. Health, physical, or mental problems

            1) Any acute physical problem such as appendicitis, viral influenza, or cancer

            2) Chronic physical problems such as lower back pain or diabetes

            3) Acute mental health problems such as mania or transient deep depression

            4) Chronic mental health problems such as schizophrenia

C. The warnings of impending stress are:

    1. Increasing dependence.

    2. Decreasing motivation, increasingly lethargic—"I am tired."

3. May become hyperalert and irritable—seems "jumpy."

4. Becomes more and more impulsive and/or impatient.

5. May have sudden outbursts of aggression, anger, or rage. This behavior is totally out of character for this individual.

6. Sleep patterns may change from 8 hours a night to 1 to 3 hours a night. This is a sign of advancing insomnia.

7. Begins to lose the ability to concentrate, even on the simplest tasks.

8. Appears "nervous."

   a. Increased pulse rate

   b. Increased blood pressure.

9. May begin to convert feelings related to stress into somatic symptoms such as headache, muscle aches, or other vague generally unmeasurable or at least difficult to measure physical signs or symptoms.

10. May lead to inability to adjust or cope effectively.

D. How to cope with stress.

1. Identify the source.

2. Relieve the stress by:

   a. Sorting out the cause(s), one element at a time.

   b. Take the day-by-day approach.

   c. If you can not change it, you will need to learn to live with it.

   d. Increase your level of physical activity.

   e. Increase your interactions with those not directly involved.

   f. Talk about the problem to those whom you believe could offer a different perspective.

   g. Balance work and play; life should not be totally one exclusive of the other.

   h. Gradually get your nutrition and sleep patterns back on track.

E. If all else fails, *get help*!

Responses to Stressors Associated With Selected Life Events.

A. Illness, both physical and mental, involving loss has the potential for a threat to self.

1. Illness involving the loss of significant aspects of life.

   a. Loss of body function

   b. Loss of body parts

   c. Loss of mobility

       d. Loss of independence

       e. Perceived impending loss of life

    2. Illness involving symptoms of mental impairment:

       a. Disorientation

       b. Confusion

       c. Hallucinations

       d. Loss of memory

B. Factors influencing an individual's reaction to illness:

    1. Family beliefs and attitudes about the cause and expected outcome of the condition

    2. Personality of the patient

    3. Anxiety expressed by the family

C. Primary defense mechanisms used by persons in dealing with illnesses or stress:

    1. Denial: Unconscious rejection of the truth.

       a. May be used by both patient and family

       b. Persistent denial may interfere with treatments offered

       c. May be used in loss of body parts, such as phantom pains after amputation

       d. Denial may promote selective hearing and induce mentally guided outcomes

       e. Becomes a limiting factor to the teaching–learning sequence

       f. Negative responses may become the normal from a previously very positive person

    2. Regression

       a. Reduces level of anxiety by returning to a less threatening and/or earlier period of life.

       b. Interests and concerns are directed at self.

       c. Generally, the behavior being exhibited is only temporary. It is used to relieve stress associated with underlying concern or problem.

       d. Early assessment of regression can lead to early intervention.

    3. Displacement

       a. Displacement in the form of anger is common.

       b. Displacement forms a barrier around the patient that can be difficult to penetrate.

       c. Can be in the form of excessive demands for attention.

       d. Overt anxiety is less acceptable than is displacing of frustration on the health care team.

       e. *Always* identify the underlying feelings.

  Other defense mechanisms include rationalization, conversion, and fantasy.

D. Changes in levels of dependence–independence functioning.

1. Independence and dependence normally coexist and are balanced. There are times in our lives when we need one of these more than the other.

2. Changes in health, even small changes, may threaten this balance.

3. Patients may feel as though they are helpless or powerless, and therefore, are more vulnerable.

    a. Patient involvement in planning care and participating in their treatments should move them toward regaining their independence.

    b. To the extent possible, patients should be allowed to choose or select from the alternatives available.

Patients should always be encouraged to function independently!

E. Grief work and closure associated with death is of great importance.

1. Types of losses:

    a. Loss of body part or function

    b. Disfigurement; substantial changes in body image, either real or imagined

    c. Loss of self-esteem, pride, and independence

    d. Loss of job, status, or financial security

    e. Loss of loved one by death or separation

    f. Impending loss of one's own life

2. Adapting to loss may include one or more of the following:

    a. Sadness and depression

    b. Anxiety

    c. Anger

    d. Guilt

    e. Helplessness

    f. Loneliness

    g. Fear

3. Kubler–Ross's five stages of the grief process are:

    a. Denial

    b. Anger

    c. Bargaining

    d. Depression

    e. Acceptance

4. If the grief process is not complete, then coping with normal life functions may be impaired.

5. Closure is the bringing to an end the feelings or thoughts about any selected event in life, and indeed life itself. For instance, closure occurs when the life cycle is completed. This includes the closure of the cycle within the group of the significant others. Life is a series of hopefully successful closures.

    a. The persons involved must be encouraged to express their feelings.

    b. Obtains reassurance with regard to those feelings.

    c. Engages in the support of the feelings of others and thereby receives support.

    d. By interactions, closure should finally be achieved.

F. Changes in body image

  1. Body image and self-concept are intimately connected.

    a. Feelings formulated by interactions with others; accepts or rejects perceived body image

    b. Internalized feelings about self formulates image

  2. Loss of body parts or function can cause a change in body image and cause one or more of the following emotions:

    a. Anxiety

    b. Denial

    c. Anger

    d. Hate

    e. Rage

    f. Depression

  3. Adaptive mechanisms in response to changes in body image may require one or more of the following:

    a. Gradual changes may be less threatening than abrupt ones.

    b. Physical or exterior changes may cause more anxiety than internal ones.

    c. Installing appropriate defense mechanisms to avoid crisis.

    d. Interactions with patient and significant others for purposes of support.

    e. Teaching both patient and significant others with regard to coping with the alteration to body image.

  4. Acceptance

    a. Is a gradual process.

    b. Intellectual acceptance occurs before emotional acceptance.

    c. Grieving brings about closure and eventually emotional acceptance.

    d. Support groups may assist with acceptance.

      1) Narcotics anonymous, NA

      2) Overeaters anonymous, OA

SEXUAL DISORDERS

Sexual disorders are divided into two groups. The first of these is *paraphilia. Para* means deviation and *philia* means that to which the person is attracted. The essential features of this group of disorders are recurrent intense sexual urges and sexually arousing fantasies generally involving (1) nonhuman objects, (2) the suffering or humiliation of oneself or one's partner (not merely simulated), or (3) children or other nonconsenting persons.

The second group of sexual disorders are the *sexual dysfunction* group. This group is characterized by inhibitions in sexual desire or the psychophysiologic changes that characterize the sexual response cycle.[2]

Paraphilia

A. Exhibitionism

1. Recurrent, intense, sexual urges and sexually arousing fantasies lasting at least 6 months.

2. Exposing one's genitals to a stranger.

3. Only found in male patients.

4. Masturbation may, or may not, accompany the act.

5. The disorder usually occurs before the age of 18, although there are indications that it may begin much later in life.

B. Fetishism

1. Recurrent, intense, sexual urges, and sexually arousing fantasies, lasting at least 6 months.

2. The sexual arousals are caused by use of nonliving objects.

3. Commonly used objects are bras, women's underpants, stocking, shoes, boots, or other wearing apparel especially undergarments.

4. The objects are held, rubbed, smelled during masturbation.

5. During sexual encounters, the person may ask his partner to wear the fetish object.

6. Without the fetish object, sexual arousal may not occur.

7. Fetish behavior usually begins in adolescence. The actual fetish will have been endowed in an earlier childhood event. The disorder tends to be chronic.

C. Frotteurism, also known as toucherism (fondling)

1. Recurrent, intense, sexual urges and sexually arousing fantasies, lasting at least 6 months.

2. Touching or rubbing against a nonconsenting person.

3. It is the touching that creates the sexual arousals, not the coercive act or the nature of the act.

4. Usually occurs in a crowded public area.

5. The disorder usually begins by adolescence.

D. Pedophilia

---

[2] DSM-III-R. 1987.

1. Recurrent, intense, sexual urges and sexually arousing fantasies, lasting at least 6 months.

2. The person acting on these urges does so with a prepubescent child.

3. The child is usually 13 or younger.

4. The pedophile is generally at least 5 years older than the child.

5. The disorder usually begins during adolescence.

E. Sexual masochism (inflicting pain on self)

1. Recurrent, intense, sexual urges and sexually arousing fantasies, lasting at least 6 months.

2. The act of sexual masochism is real.

3. Involves being humiliated, beaten, bound, or using other techniques to create suffering

4. These masochistic fantasies are likely to have been present in childhood.

5. The fantasy becomes reality.

F. Sexual sadism (inflicting pain on others)

1. Recurrent, intense, sexual urges and sexually arousing fantasies, lasting at least 6 months.

2. This disorder involves real acts in which psychological or physical suffering of the victim is sexually arousing.

3. Sexual sadism is likely to have been present in childhood.

G. Transvestic fetishism

1. Recurrent, intense, sexual urges and sexually arousing fantasies, lasting at least 6 months.

2. Cross-dressing, that is the dressing in the apparel of the opposite sex.

3. May begin in childhood or early adolescence.

H. Voyeurism

1. Recurrent, intense, sexual urges and sexually arousing fantasies, lasting at least 6 months.

2. Involves the act of observing unsuspecting people, usually strangers, who are either naked, in the process of disrobing, or engaged in sexual activity.

3. Formerly known as "peeping Tom."

4. Usual onset is before age 15.

Sexual Dysfunction—The Sexual Response Cycle

A. Appetitive: Involves fantasies about sexual activity accompanied by the desire to have sex by both men and women

B. Excitement: Subjective sense of sexual pleasure accompanied by physiologic changes in both men and women.

C. Orgasm: The peaking of sexual pleasure, with release of sexual tension and rhythmic contraction of the perineal muscles and pelvic reproductive organs in the female. In the male, it is the inevitable release of semen and sperm that is also associated with the rhythmic contraction of the urethra.

D. Resolution: This phase of the cycle consists of a sense of general relaxation, wellbeing, and muscular relaxation. Sexual dysfunctions may be psychogenic (originate in the mind) and/or biogenic (originating in the genetics of the body).

E. Sexual desire disorders

F. Sexual arousal disorders

G. Orgasm disorders

H. Sexual pain disorders[3]

SUMMARY

The key points in Chapter 1 that are most likely to occur in the NCLEX-PN examination are:

- Personality
- Personality development
- Freud
- Erickson
- Defense mechanisms (**important for Boards**)

Review Questions

1. According to Freudian theory, which of the following is the most primitive component of the personality?

    a. Id.
    b. Ego.
    c. Superego.
    d. Libido.

2. A person who always has an excuse is:

    a. Immature.
    b. Rationalizing.
    c. Fantasizing.
    d. In passive withdrawal.

3. The mechanism by which a primitive or unacceptable tendency or behavior is redirected into socially constructive channels is known as:

    a. Regression.
    b. Sublimation.

---

[3] Adapted from DSM-III-R, 1987.

c. Rationalization.

d. Suppression.

4. A male child is demonstrating the Oedipus complex. Which of the following is the source of attraction?

a. Cats.

b. Mother.

c. Father.

d. Sexual peers.

5. Mr. Green tells the nurse, "the voices tell me I am wicked and that I must be punished." Which of the following is your BEST response?

a. "Don't be silly, there are no voices."

b. "What you hear must be very frightening, can you tell me about the voices."

c. "If you are going to talk about voices, I am leaving."

d. "People around here hear voices all the time, how are your voices different?"

6. According to Freud, which of the following mediate between the other two personality components?

a. Ego.

b. Id.

c. Superego.

d. Complex.

7. Prevention of dangerous feelings and desires from being expressed by exaggeration of the opposite attitude or behavior is which of the following?

a. Projection.

b. Displacement.

c. Reaction–formation.

d. Repression.

8. Expending energy to remove internalized feelings from one person to someone who is nearby and less threatening is known as:

a. Perception.

b. Projection.

c. Displacement.

d. Silly.

9. Regression may be used as a defense mechanism to meet the patient's need for:

a. Safety and security.

b. Self-actualization.

c. Love and belonging.

d. Power and control.

10. Self-recognition that "I am not very good when I work with numbers, but I am great when I work with languages" is an example of which of the following:

a. Displacement.

b. Projection.

c. Compensation.

d. Identification.

CHAPTER 2

Review of Therapeutic Communication

KEY CHAPTER OBJECTIVES

Upon completion of Chapter 2, the student should be able to:

- Identify all threats, put-downs and judgmental statements as not therapeutic regardless of whether written or verbal.
- Be able to use therapeutic communications in verbal interactions with patients, coworkers, and others.
- Identify therapeutic communication.

REVIEW OF THERAPEUTIC COMMUNICATION

The key concept in this chapter is: if any statement or action contains a threat, a judgment, or a put-down, it is not therapeutic.

Always go for the underlying feeling. What you see is not necessarily reflecting the true or underlying feeling. You will need to interact with the patient in order to understand the underlying feeling. These feelings are always guarded by the patient. The deeper the feelings, the longer it will take to get at them. Always go for the underlying feeling. Emotions are somewhat like onions. You must peel layer after layer to arrive at the real feeling.

Therapeutic communication is effective and purposeful communication between individuals, more specifically between health professionals (nurse) and the patient.

PURPOSE(S) OF THERAPEUTIC COMMUNICATION

A. Obtain useful information.

B. Maintain or develop a healthy personal relationship.

C. Identify current or potential health problems.

D. Examine resources for coping.

E. Assist the patient with developing defense mechanisms.

F. Teach problem solving techniques.

G. Identify patient strengths or assets.

The Basis for Therapeutic Communications

A. Sensitivity

    1. Ability to listen and learn by observing.

    2. Assure patients that their need to be heard will be respected.

B. Trust

    1 Welcoming by name, and escort in an unhurried manner.

    2. Introduction to other staff members.

    3. All information collected is confidential.

C. Listening attentively.

D. Willingness to greet and offer self.

E. Provide a sounding board.

F. No threats, judgments, no put-downs.

BASIC CONCEPTS OF THERAPEUTIC COMMUNICATION

A. Clarify your ideas before communicating.

B. Examine carefully the true purpose of each communication.

C. Consider the total physical and human setting whenever you communicate.

D. Consult with others, when appropriate, in planning communications.

E. Be sensitive, during communication, especially to the overtness as well as the basic content of your message.

F. If the opportunity arises, convey something of meaning and value to the receiver.

G. Follow-up your communication.

H. Communicate for tomorrow as well as today.

I. Be certain that your behavior is consistent with your message.

J. Communication is a two way process, strive to be understood as well as to understand.

K. *Be objective—never subjective.*

Foundations of Interpersonal Communication

A. Nurses must understand how strongly their behavior influences interactions with others.

B. Nurses and patients bring expectations to the interaction. This isn't a one-way message.

    1. Nurses must learn to *accept* differences between individuals.

    2. Differences may be life style, social values, cultural diversity, etc.

    3. You do not and indeed are not expected to buy into the difference in values — simply accept it.

C. Mental health staff must strive to use the collaborative process to assess patients for strengths, weaknesses, goals, and insightfulness.

Note: *Weaknesses are now known as areas for improvement.*

    1. Communication must be clear!

    2. Communication may be selectively different from patient to patient, but *at all times* communication must be therapeutic.

    3. Nurses are most effective when they are in the position of understanding the total plan of care for each patient.

    4. Nurses are valuable contributors to the plan of care as they most frequently communicate with the patient.

    5. Without effective collaborative communication, the united front is weakened, the milieu threatened, and the increased possibility of patient manipulation of both staff and milieu.

6. All humans have selective hearing, that is, they filter out what they choose *not* to hear. In the mental health setting, selective hearing can be carried to extremes from staff splitting to the incorporation of the spoken word into the delusional system of the patient. *Be certain that rules, guidelines, and other written materials are reflected in a consistent and organized milieu.*

D. Communication is essential in the continuity of care, in terms of discharge planning, agency referrals, and in working with the family members.

Reasons for Ineffective Communication

A. Erroneous message sent: The sender did not say what was intended to be said.

B. Selective hearing: Receiver *only* heard what he/she chose to hear.

C. Verbal and nonverbal messages confuse the receiver by not agreeing.

D. The message was covert.

E. Communication lost when language interpreted by receiver. This is attributed to word(s) misinterpreted because the message could have more than one meaning.

F. The message contained many generalities when specifics were expected and needed, hence confusion results.

G. Avoid double binds (saying one thing and doing the opposite of what is said).

H. Being involved in triangulation.

DEFINITION

TRIANGULATION: Engaging in a three way miscommunication. None of the three parties understand fully, nor could any of them fully comply with the message content. Any one of the three persons may become the scapegoat of the communication.

Blocks to Effective Communication

A. Threats

B. Judgments

C. Put-downs

D. Defensive statements used to repel verbal attack.

E. Stereotypical statements—insensitive.

F. Avoidance: a different topic will derail a topic that causes anxiety.

G. Insincerity in any of its many forms.

H. Glibness or superficiality.

I. Making inflammatory statements or any other kind of statement that causes defenses to go up to protect the self. This may be the perception that an inflammatory statement was made during the conversation.

J. Using terse (offensive) verbal comments.

Most effective techniques of communication are based on the following nurse qualities:

1. Patience

2. Persistence

3. Tactfulness

4. Ingenuity

5. Sincerity

6. Honesty

A. Validating statements that affirm perceptions by nurse.

B. Clarifying statements that serve to dispel misunderstanding or requests for additional information that would lead to a better understanding.

C. Open-ended (broad) questions that permit the patient to discuss topics of their choice.

D. Reflecting statements: ascertain that the statement made has been correctly received.

E. Confrontational statements: A direct verbal assault on the patient's belief to cause rethinking of the belief or idea in question. This requires skill to provide a confrontation that is therapeutic rather than a verbal assault.

SUMMARY

Effective techniques: the most important concept is that if the statement is threatening, judgmental or, contains a put-down, then it is not therapeutic.

Review Questions

To pass the NCLEX it is critical that you understand therapeutic communications. The NCLEX questions are designed to (1) ascertain that you are *safe* to practice at the entry Practical/Vocational level and)2 that you can correctly identify the *most* therapeutic answer. Here are some sample questions for you to review.

1. A patient tells you, in no uncertain terms, that he/she is upset by the inability of the staff to meet her/his needs because the staff is "stupid". He/she appears agitated, angry and is uncooperative. The most therapeutic response you can make is:

    a. "If this behavior continues, we will have to take you to seclusion."
    b. It is time for you to calm down."
    c. Everyone here is trying to help you. Please try to help yourself."
    d. I have some time, can you tell me about the reason for your anger."

2. Which of the following communications is the most therapeutic when a patient is crying and pacing the floor.

a. Let me help you".
b. "If I had more time, I could help you."
c. "You need a tranquilizer".
d. "May I stay with you until you can tell me what is wrong?"

3. A patient is sitting in the day room and appears to be quietly talking to her/him-self. Which of the following would be most therapeutic?

a. "Can you tell me why you are talking to yourself?"
b. "Would you please quit talking to yourself, I have something to tell you."
c. "I can see that you are talking." "May I listen in."
d. "If you have something to say, I am here, and I will listen to you."

4. During the admission process, a patient that you are interviewing and talking with suddenly says "I have told everyone the same answers at least three times, are you cross checking my answers with the rest of the staff? Your most therapeutic response would be:

a. "No, I just want to hear it for myself."
b. "Sometimes the questions are repeated, we are trying to learn about you so we can help".
c. "Does it seem to you that I am being nosy?"
d. "Yes, we always check out the stories that patients tell us."

5. A patient tells you that he/she is depressed because of a recent death in the family. Which of the following is most therapeutic?

a. "If you would like to talk about your feelings about death, I will listen".
b. "Let's talk about something else."
c. "I can relate to that, someone in my family just died."
d. "Death is a very difficult subject to discuss."

6. The most therapeutic approach in dealing with the patient who is in denial is to:

a. Leave them alone.
b. Aggressively confront the denial.
c. Be matter of fact and reinforce reality.
d. Offer alternative activities.

7. A patient says "if I were not so depressed I would kill myself." Your response would be:

a. "Can you tell me more about your depression?"
b. "Can you tell me how you would kill yourself?"
c. "You really do seem depressed."
d. "Why would you want to kill yourself?"

8. To use verbal therapeutic communication most effectively, you would avoid which of the following during therapeutic communication?

a. Asking only "yes" or "no" questions.
b. Asking open ended questions.
c. Asking questions that are related only to the discussion.
d. Asking questions that are clear and concise, but that generally include the need for the patient to discuss in detail.

9. Sometimes during patient – staff interactions it becomes necessary for the patient to reflect on the questions that have been asked. When there is a pause in the communication, it is best to:

   a. Leave, let her/him think it over.
   b. Sit quietly by, until the patient is ready to continue.
   c. Press for an answer to the question.
   d. Tell her/him that they will have to answer more quickly, you have things to do.

10. When making initial contact with a patient, it is most important to remember that:

   a. The patient is used to being locked in a hospital.
   b. Hostile patients are the result of hostile staff.
   c. At this point, both staff and patient are strangers to one another.
   d. You should be therapeutic, as first impressions are important to patients.

CHAPTER 3

Admitting to the Mental Health Setting

KEY CHAPTER OBJECTIVES

Upon completion of Chapter 3, the student should be able to identify satisfactorily correct answers to questions regarding the following knowledge areas:

- Admissions—define each of the following:
    1. Voluntary
    2. Involuntary
    3. Commitment
    4. Emergency admissions
    5. Patients' rights
    6. Confidentiality
    7. Advance directives
- Assist with the physical examination—a review.
- Assist with the mental status examination.
- Be able to identify the key components of the mental status examination.
- Be able to assist with implementing additional nursing considerations at the time of admission.
- Be able to document observations.

TYPES OF ADMISSIONS

The admission of a patient to a mental health facility occurs as a two-part process. The first part is the establishment of the need to be hospitalized. This is based on the assessment of the psychiatrist. The continuation of the first part is the actual admission procedure to the hospital. The patient must undergo the rigors of verifying essential biographical data such as name, address, and place of residence. During this interviewing process, eligibility for care is established. Following these preliminary steps, the admission documents are signed and witnessed by the appropriate admissions staff.

The second part of the admission begins with the nursing staff on the various nursing units to which the patient has been admitted.

Admission of the Patient to Acute Care

Voluntary

A. Patient agrees to admission.

B. Patient willingly signs Authorization for Treatment.

C. Patient recognizes need for hospitalization.

D. Patient has choice of program (chemical dependency, psychiatry, etc.).

E. Patient usually has been under the care of a psychiatrist or other mental health professional.

Involuntary

Each of the states has established legal criteria for admission. Generally speaking, the guidelines for involuntary admission are: presents a serious harm to self or others (suicidal or homicidal) or harm may be demonstrated either by the person's behavior or by evidence of severe emotional distress and deterioration in her/his mental condition to the extent that the person cannot remain at liberty and requires treatment.

Involuntary admissions are arranged by one (or more) of the following:

A. Emergency Detention (ED) Warrant—an application is filed, generally at the Mental Health Department, by a family member or an officer of the law.

B. Types of applications for treatment are temporary commitment for mental illness, court-ordered treatment for alcoholism, and court-ordered treatment for drug dependency.

Once the warrant is issued, the patient will be held at the treatment facility, usually for 24 hours or whatever the time frame specified in the warrant. This is known as involuntary emergency admission (IEA). This is done to permit professionals time to assess the patient for the need to treat.

A. Order of protective custody (OPC) is filed in the court in conjunction with an application for court ordered mental health services and a certificate of medical examination for mental illness issued by a physician who has examined the patient within the previous 5 days. The OPC authorizes the hospital to detain the patient for up to 72 hours pending the probable cause hearing.

B. Commitment is based on the findings of the court. The judge may order the person committed for a period up to 12 months for treatment. The judge may also order inpatient or outpatient care, or dismiss the case.

C. Patients under 16 years of age may be admitted involuntarily with consent of parents or by court order.

Check your state's legal policy and procedure for commitment.

PATIENTS' RIGHTS

Patients do not give up any rights by being admitted to a hospital for mental health treatment. Under no circumstance may a patient be held against his/her will!! Patients do have the following rights as defined by Federal Law:

A. All of the rights of any citizen of the United States.

B. The right of habeas corpus—patients have the right to ask a judge if it is legal to be kept in the hospital.

C. The patients retain the rights of property, guardianship, family, religion, the right to register and vote, sue and be sued, sign contracts, and all other rights related to licenses, permits, privileges, and benefits under the law.

D. The patients are presumed mentally competent unless a court has ruled otherwise.

E. The right to a clean and humane environment, protected from harm; to be provided privacy with regards to personal needs and to be treated with respect and dignity.

F. The right to appropriate treatment in the most open place available that provides protection for both patients and the persons around them.

G. To be free from mistreatment, abuse, neglect, and exploitation.

H. The patients must know *in advance* the cost of services, sources of reimbursement, and any limits on length of service.

I. If patients provide a service for the facility then they are entitled to "fair compensation" in accordance with the Fair Labor Standards Act.

J. Before admission to the hospital, patients have the right to be informed of *all* hospital rules and regulations regarding the conduct and course of the program of treatment.

K. The right to communicate:

1. Talk to people outside of the hospital.

2. Write to people outside of the hospital.

3. Send and receive sealed and uncensored mail.

4. Limits may be set on certain of these rights, but if limits are set then:

a. Extent of limits must be written in the medical record, signed by the physician, dated, and contain the nature of the limit.

b. Must be reviewed at least every 7 days; review outcome must appear in writing.

c. The patient may contact her/his attorney or the attorney may contact her/his patient-client.

L. The patients may refuse to take part in research.

M. The patients may refuse any of the following:

1. Surgical procedures

2. Electroconvulsive therapy

3. Unusual medications

4. Hazardous assessment procedures

5. Use of audiovisual equipment that would record behavior

6. Any other procedures for which permission is required by law

N. The right to revoke permission at any time although a previous permission had been given.

Rights Related to Care and Treatment

A. The patients have a right to an individualized plan of treatment.

1. The patients have the right to take part in developing their treatment plan.

2. The patients have the right to take part (and should) in developing the discharge treatment plan for care, both during the inpatient phase and after leaving the hospital.

3. These rights are extended to parents or other legal guardians in the case of a minor.

4. Patients may request that parent(s) or legal guardians be included in the preparation of the inpatient as well as outpatient treatment plans.

B. The patients must have full disclosure of all care, procedures, and treatments that they will be given. The disclosures need to include the following elements:

1. Risks

2. Side effects

3. Benefits of medications and treatments

4. If the treatments or medications are:

a. Unusual

b. Experimental

c. Other treatment alternatives

5. The consequences of refusing the prescribed treatment(s)

C. Patients may refuse medications if:

1. They don't want them.

2. They don't need them.

3. They feel it is too much.

4. The medication is mood and/or mind-altering.

D. The exception to patients refusing their medications is that the right to refuse has been specifically taken away by court order.

E. The patients may not be physically restrained unless specifically ordered by the physician in the medical record. If patients are physically restrained, they must know the reason, how long they will be restrained, and exactly the behavior that is expected to be removed from physical restraint. The least restrictive form of restraint must be used. Verbal interventions are the least restrictive, and physical restraints are the most restrictive.

F. The patients have the right to meet with the staff who is responsible for their care and to be told of the staff's professional discipline, job title, and responsibilities. Also the patients have the right to know about any proposed change in the appointment of staff, professional, or otherwise who is directly responsible for their care.

G. The patients have the right to a second opinion by another physician at the patients' expense.

H. The patients have the right to know why they are being transferred to another program within the hospital or outside the hospital.

Special Rights Granted to Voluntary Patients

Among these are:

A. Patients have the right to leave the hospital* within a legally predetermined period to time after they have informed the staff verbally or in writing that they choose to leave. If the patient tells a staff person but does not write it down, then the staff is required to write the request for the patient.

B. There are only three reasons that the patient would not be allowed to leave within the time frame specified as the waiting period:

1. If the patient changes his/her mind and decide to stay.

2. If the physician believes that a longer stay is required for psychiatric reasons (either the patient wants to kills him/herself or wants to kill someone else and has an active plan), then the physician applies for court-ordered services or an emergency detention is filed with a judge. The judge is asked to decide whether or not further psychiatric services are needed. The application must be filed with the court during the time frame of the waiting period.

3. If the patient is under the age of 16 and the person who admitted the patient does not want the patient to leave. Parent(s) or legal guardian(s) may communicate with the physician and provide the hospital with a written and signed statement that the patient should not leave.

C. Within the time frame set by law of requesting to leave the hospital, the patient must be examined face-to-face by the physician and a determination has to be made whether or not the patient is ready to be discharged. The results of the assessment must be documented in the medical record indicating whether or not the physician intends to apply for court-ordered treatment. If the physician determines that the patient is ready to be discharged, then the discharge must occur without any further delay.

D. Commitment of the voluntarily admitted patient can only occur under the two following conditions:

1. The physician determines that the patient needs continued treatment, and the patient has left the hospital without asking permission.

2. The physician determines that continued treatment is essential and the patient refuses treatment or the patient is unable to agree to further treatment.

Special Rights of Patients Apprehended for Emergency Detention [those brought to the hospital against their will but with legal (judge) permission.]

A. Patients have the right to be told:

1. Where they are.

2. Why they are being held.

3. That they may be held for a longer time if the judge decides its in their best interest.

4. They have the right to call a lawyer. Assistance in calling the lawyer must be given if staff is ask to call the lawyer for the patient.

5. They have the right to be seen by a physician prior to admission.

a. The physician decides whether or not the patient is likely to do harm to self or to others. If the physician determines that the patient is harmful to self or others, then he/she obtains an ED from legal authority.

b. Or the physician may determine that the mental condition is worsening.

c. If patients are detained, they must be told that they have a right to a hearing for that detention within a specified time frames, for example, 72 hours. The maximum period of detention is set by state law, for example, 24 hours.

d. If the patients are not to be detained, then efforts will be made to return them to where they came.

e. The patients must also be notified that anything they say or do may be used in proceedings for further detention.

Special Rights of Persons Held on Order of Protective Custody

A. The patients have the right to call an attorney.

B. Before a probable cause hearing (probable means to establish if there is sufficient reason to proceed) to determine whether or not the patients are to be detained, they must be told in writing that:

1. They have been placed under an order of protective custody.

2. Why the order was issued.

3. The date, time, and place of hearing to determine whether or not they must remain in custody until the hearing.

4. This notice must also be given to the patients' attorney.

C. The patients' hearing must occur within the legally established time frame, for example, 72 hours.

D. The patients must be released from custody according to the following criteria:

1. If the time frame has elapsed and the hearing has not occurred.

2. The court has not issued an order for mental health services within 14 days of an application.

3. The physician finds that the patient no longer needs court-ordered mental health services.

CONFIDENTIALITY—ANOTHER RIGHT

A. The patients have the right to review the information contained in the medical record. This right is extended to parents and legal guardians in the case of minors. In the case of legal incompetence, the court has access to medical records.

B. The patients have the right to have their records kept private and to be told about the conditions under which information about them can be revealed without the patients' express written consent.

C. The patients have the right to be informed of the current and future use of products of special observation and audiovisual techniques, such as one-way vision mirrors, tape recorders, television, movies, or photographs.

Advance Directives for All Patients

Federal law requires that all patients be given information regarding their right to health care decisions in advance. By giving advance directives, the patient can tell the doctor and family about the medical care that the patient would choose to receive and whether or not the patient would choose to have another person make the decisions in the event the patient was no longer able to make decisions for her/himself.

The patient may (but is not required) to leave advance directives about life support in the event of terminal illness. This is often termed a "directive to physicians" or as a "living will". A Directive to Physicians tells your physician and family about the types of life support that you want to be provided or withheld in the event you become terminally ill and are no longer able to make decisions.

The patient may designate person(s) to make medical treatment decisions for him/her by naming someone to have a "durable power of attorney for health care.". Should a durable power of attorney be in force the person named will be able to choose health-care alternatives for the patient should the doctor decide that the patient is no longer able to make his/her own decisions.

The durable power of attorney for health care applies to all health care-decisions including decisions to withhold or withdraw life-sustaining systems in the event of terminal illness.

The directive to physicians is an advance directive that deals only with terminal illness and the withholding or withdrawal of life-sustaining procedures. If the patient already has either a directive to physician, or a durable power of attorney for health care, the hospital needs a copy of the document for inclusion in the medical record where it would be available for the health-care staff.

> Should the physician caring for the patient have reservations or concerns about the advance directive, then the patient and the physician should strive to resolve these concerns. Should the physician and the patient not agree, the matter may be referred to the patient advocate, ethics committee, or to other appropriate arbitration.

All hospitals require that a patient sign a statement indicating whether or not an advance directive is in force. Should an advance directive be needed at a later time in the hospitalization, it can be done either verbally to the physician in the presence of two witnesses or in writing by an attorney of the patient's choice.

If an advance directive is in force it should be placed in the active patient chart in a conspicuous place, i.e., with signed treatment authorizations.

Just one more item concerning advance directives: the patient may use the advance directives to allow the staff to medicate or otherwise manage out-of-control behavior. By giving advance notice, the staff can administer one dose of the PRN medications regardless of what the patient says about it at the time of the out-of-control behavior.

Advance directives are not limited to such issues as life support, but may be linked directly to the care received during mental health treatment.

ASSESSMENT

A thorough physical examination and a detailed assessment of mental processes should be accomplished, unless otherwise specified, within 8 hours of admission for all patients. These two examinations are integrated and areas of concern, physical or mental (emotional), are identified. Once the physical and/or mental problems are identified, then a preliminary treatment plan can be opened. The preliminary and master treatment plans are forms that everyone on the team can and should contribute to.

The following is optional and is intended for those who are in need of a review of physical assessment. Generally, the registered nurse is responsible for the completion of the physical examination. You should be familiar with some of the basic elements of the examination, which are listed here.

Elements of the Physical Examination (PE)

Physical examinations are ordinarily accomplished from head to toe, right to left, front and back. The PE is a systematic and sequential evaluation of not only physiologic systems, but mental status as well.

Since you may be examining either adults or children, you will need to keep in mind basic differences in physiology and anatomy and vary your assessment accordingly. For instance, taking an adult blood pressure (BP) requires a BP cuff of appropriate size. Remember that a child's BP cuff will also vary according to size of patient. This is only one example of adapting to patient's need.

Ordinarily, the PN/VN, whether student or licensed, will be responsible for a set of baseline vital signs, which will include at least the following: an accurate BP, temperature, pulse, respiration, height, and weight. Usually a vision screening is also completed; the Snellen chart is a commonly used vision examination.

Using the principles of inspection, palpation, percussion, and auscultation, the physical includes at least the following:

A. Skin or integumentary system

   1. Color

   2. Texture

   3. Unusual growths, hair, moles

   4. Moisture; dry, wet

   5. Temperature of skin

   6. Finger and toe nails

B. Head

   1. Skull

   2. Scalp

   3. Face

   4. Eyes

   5. Nose

   6. Ears

   7. Mouth

   8. Neck, including throat

   9. The skin is included in all components of the physical examination.

C. Chest or thorax

   1. Respirations (right and left, front and back)

   2. Cardiovascular (right and left, front and back) may include obtaining an electrocardiogram

   3. Breasts and axilla (right and left)

D. Upper extremities (right and left)

   1. Skin surfaces

   2. Moisture content, dry or moist

   3. Color

    4. Pulses

E. Abdominal examination (front and back, right and left, perineal) includes gastrointestinal and skin examinations

    1. General appearance; scars, surgical

    2. Assess dietary habits

    3. Elimination

    4. Changes in dietary and/or elimination functions

F. Urinary functioning

G. Reproductive functioning

H. Musculoskeletal functioning

I. Neurological functioning

J. Endocrine functioning

K. Immune functioning

    These are the essentials contained in a physical assessment.

    Remember: Check local admission policy and procedures at your clinical facility.

    The following are the key assessment elements contained in the psychiatric or mental health survey. During the admission process of the mental health patient, the emphasis is on the components listed:

A. General appearance

    1. Grooming

    2. Neat

    3. Well-groomed

    4. Unkempt

    5. Dress, describe in detail

    6. Posture

        a. Erect

        b. Rigid

        c. Relaxed

        d. Other

B. Orientation

    1. Time

    2. Place

    3. Person

    4. Why are you here?

C. Speech

    1. Speed

    2. Volume

    3. Quantity

    4. Pace

     5. Pressured

     6. Diction

     7. Relevant

     8. Content

     9. Clarity

     10. Sequential

     11. Organized

     12. Coherent

D. Eyes

     1. Contact

        a. Good

        b. Minimal

        c. None

     2. Pupils — see physical

E. Attitude (mood or affect)

     1. Resistive

     2. Cooperative

     3. Self-depreciative

     4. Suspicious

     5. Trusting

     6. Depressed

     7. Aloof

     8. Assaultive

     9. Fearful

     10. Tearful

F. Mood — let the patients describe their mood. How do you feel?

G. Affect; what kind of behavior does the patient exhibit? How does he/she react to her/his surroundings?

     1. Flat

     2. Labile

     3. Blunted

     4. Sad

     5. Elated

     6. Euphoric

     7. Angry

     8. Laughing

H. Thought processes

1. Oriented to reality
2. Talkative
3. Hesitant
4. Repetitious
5. Monosyllabic
6. Mute
7. Evasive
8. Reluctant
9. Flight of ideas
10. Disconnected thoughts
11. Illogical sequence
12. Loose associations
13. Rapid thoughts
14. Organized or
15. Disorganized
16. Easily distracted
17. Blocking
18. Echolalia
19. Perseveration

I. Thought contents: if yes to any of these, quote what the patient has to say about them.

1. Hallucinations
   a. Visual
   b. Auditory
   c. Tactile
   d. Olfactory
2. Obsessions
   a. Present
   b. Not present
3. Phobias
   a. Yes
   b. No
4. Illusions
   a. Yes
   b. No
5. Ideas of reference
   a. Yes

          b. No

     6. Delusions, yes or no

          a. If yes, what type?

          b. Grandeur

          c. Somatic

          d. Persecutory

     7. Perception of the current situation

     8. Psychomotor responses

          a. Slow

          b. Fast

          c. Coordinated

          d. Restless

          e. Uncoordinated

          f. Agitated

          g. Pacing

          h. Tics

          i. Tremulous

          j. Other responses

     9. Memory

          a. Intact

          b. Recent

          c. Remote (ability to retain by listening)

          d. Recall

   10. Intelligence

   11. Judgment

          a. Good

          b. Fair

          c. Poor

          d. Based on decisions

   12. Insightfulness

          a. Understanding of what caused the problem

          b. Not sure what caused the problem

          c. Is unaware of a problem

J. Suicide assessment — key questions to be asked

     1. Are you now or have you ever thought seriously about killing yourself?

          a. If yes — Do you have a plan?

          b. If yes — What is your plan?

    c. After the plan is detailed — Give me the (object) with which you intend to harm yourself.

    d. Contract — if you experience thoughts of hurting (killing) yourself, will you let one of the staff know?

K. Homicide assessment

  1. Do you now or have you ever wanted to kill someone else?

  2. Who is the person you want to kill?

  3. Do you have a plan?

Additional Nursing Considerations on Admission

A safe milieu is of primary importance. What follows is an outline of safety measures considered on admission and these should provide a safe milieu.

A. A physical search of the patient (if ordered).

B. A search of the patient's belongings (with written consent) .There must be a consent.

C. A listing of the patient's personal belongings.

D. Searches are conducted to identify and to remove the following items:

  1. Sharp objects

  2. Flammable substances — perfumes, hair sprays, etc.

  3. Belts, ropes, any material that could be made into a suicide device

  4. All medications

  5. Any other items found on the unit or on patient such as:

    a. Knives—all metal objects, i.e., keys

    b. Tools

    c. Aerosol spray cans

    d. Electric blankets

    e. Anything with an electric cord

    f. Electric hot plates or any object that generates enough heat to injure flesh

    g. Cleaners or solvents

    h. Cameras

    i. Tape recorders

    j. Glass items (especially compacts)

    k. Razor blades

    l. Razors with blades

    m. Mirrors — any item that shatters and causes smaller pieces with sharp edges. Even plastic credit cards will cut skin quite easily

      n. Scissors

  6. Other items subject to appropriateness of milieu such as:

    a. Posters related to death or satanism

    b. Drawings of questionable content

    c. Wearing apparel that refers to

      1. Drugs

      2. Alcohol

      3. Sexual topics

      4. Violence (in any form)

      5. Bondage

      6. Profanity

      7. Satanism or satanic worship

      8. Themes of satanism

      9. References to the occult

      10. Death

E. Searches of the patient's area may be done at any time, with permission of the patient, with the patient present during the search, and with physician order.

F. Searches are conducted by staff of the same gender as the patient.

G. Sharps are stored in non-patient areas under lock.

Nursing Staff must be continually alert for any addition of dangerous materials to the milieu. Patients must know that searches will or could be done upon completion of therapeutic passes if ordered by the doctor.

Patient Orientation to the Milieu

A. Tour of the nursing unit

B. The patient should receive an information packet

C. The patient should become familiar with fire escape routes

D. Introduction to staff

E. Any other specific information as appropriate

Differences in the various milieu will be discussed as a part of each chapter.

NURSING PROCESS

Now that all the information is assembled from the physical assessment and the mental status assessment, it will be necessary to organize it in an acceptable format.

Any one of many formats is possible. Regardless of the format, the following components must appear: assessment, planning, implementing, and evaluation.

APIE

A = assessment. This component has two parts: *subjective* and *objective*.

The subjective component consists of the patient statements, in quotes or from the person (family or significant other) being interviewed. These subjective responses should be appropriate and reflect organized and consistent thought patterns. Statements such as "I am going to kill myself" should alert staff that immediate action needs to be taken. The exact intervention is directed by the appropriate follow-up questions.

Objective means observed. These are measures that are both observable and measurable to staff conducting the assessment. Blood pressures and temperature are observable and measurable and therefore, objective.

The *assessment* is summarization of the subjective and the objective data. For example, if the subjective statement is "I am going to kill myself" and the objective data reflects lacerations with bleeding on left and right wrists, then the assessment is a suicidal act of self-mutilation. This is then termed a problem to be resolved.

P = plan or strategy for solving the problem. How would you proceed with the plan? First, you know that the patient has made a choice to commit suicide. You would pursue a contract, either verbal or written, that if the patient feels a strong threat to self that he/she will immediately notify staff. Second, you would want to closely observe the patient for any further self-destructive behavior (checks every 15 minutes). Third, you will need to talk to the patient to try to find an underlying cause that has motivated the suicidal behavior.

I = implementation, interventions; remember that these interventions are based on the A(ssessment) and the P(lan).

A. A written or verbal contract with the patients that they will immediately notify staff if they have the uncontrollable urge to hurt themselves.

B. Check on the patients every 15 minutes for safety's sake. A one nurse – one patient or 1:1 is the most appropriate approach to managing a suicidal patient who has an active plan.

C. Talk (verbal intervention) with the patient to try to determine the underlying cause of the suicidal thoughts and gestures.

E = evaluation. After the implementation, you will need to know if the plan is effective. If the plan is working, then it will be continued until it is no longer needed. If the plan is not working, then the evaluation should reflect the need to alter or modify the plan. In this case, if the patient states that he/she no longer has thoughts of committing suicide, then the problem is solved. However, if the suicidal thinking continues then the plan and subsequently the implementation may need to be revised to meet the immediate safety needs of the patient.

This is the SOAPE (subjective, objective, assessment, plan, and evaluation) format of the nursing process. It is quite easy to construct a plan for the return to good mental health if you have sufficient data.

BIRP Charting

Another way to chart or plan is called the BIRP format.

B = behavior.
I = intervention.
R = response.
P = plan.

BIRP charting addresses the issues of behavior, as behavior is generally the most observable activity in the mental health milieu. In this case, you would identify a behavior (usually unacceptable) and plan an appropriate intervention to correct, modify, or alter it.

After the intervention, there will usually be a response to the intervention, such as the patient no longer has suicidal ideation. Then the plan component would be directed at maintaining or monitoring the behavior for future intervention.

During your learning/clinical experience, you may see other forms of charting. Those forms will most likely contain the elements of the APIE, BIRP, or SOAPE formats.

SUMMARY

The important concepts to be reviewed in this chapter are: voluntary and involuntary admissions, the elements of commitment, emergency admissions, and all of these as they are related to patients' rights, confidentiality, and advance directives. This chapter also contains a review of physical examinations, mental status, and nursing documentation using APIE, SOAPE, and BIRP formats.

Review Questions

1. A voluntary admission is one that:
   a. The patient has requested by signing the admission forms.
   b. The patient has not requested, but that is required and enforced by law.
   c. The patient's family has demanded because of inappropriate behavior on the part of the patient.
   d. The judge ordered the hospitalization.

2. An involuntary admission is one that:
   a. The patient has requested.
   b. The judge has ordered the hospitalization.
   c. Is an order of protective custody.
   d. Required by law.

3. The A in APIE stands for:
   a. Admission.
   b. Appendectomy.
   c. Assessment.
   d. Association.

4. An example of an objective measurement is:

   a. Fever.
   b. Pain.
   c. Vital signs. .
   d. Feelings.

5. An example of a subjective measurement is:

   a. Blood pressure.
   b. "I feel bad." .
   c. Temperature.
   d. Pulse pressure.

6. An example of a plan statement would be:

   a. "Will feel better."
   b. "Will take pills."
   c. "Will contact a staff member immediately if feelings or thoughts of suicide become overwhelming."·
   d. "Will attend activities as scheduled."

7. An example of an evaluation statement would be:

   a. "Feels better."
   b. "Suicidal thoughts are gone.".
   c. "Attends most activities."
   d. "Wants to leave."

8. Objective statements are made based on:

   a. A direct quote from the patient as to his/her current feelings or thoughts.
   b. Measurable, observable data collected from patient.
   c. How the nurse feels about the situation.
   d. Staff statements about the way the patient is behaving.

9. Subjective statements found in the nursing care plan are:

   a. Statements from the patient. ·
   b. Statements made by staff persons who are unable to assess the patient's needs or feelings.
   c. Measurable and observable data only.
   d. Statements made by the patient that are relevant to the plan of care.

10. Together, the subjective and objective components of data collection form what is known as:

    a. Assessment.
    b. Association.
    c. Apathy.
    d. Analysis

Dealing with Life-Threatening Crisis

KEY CHAPTER OBJECTIVES

Upon completion of Chapter 4, the student should be able to identify satisfactorily correct answers to questions regarding the following knowledge areas:

The student will be able to recognize a life-threatening crisis.

The student will be able to:

- Assist in identifying persons who are suicidal.
- Assist with an appropriate suicide intervention.
- Assist with the care of a person who has posttraumatic stress disorder.
- Assist in identifying violent behavior.
- Assist with the rape victim.
- Assist with the incest victim.
- Assist with the management of the patient who is exhibiting aggressive behavior.
- Assist with the patient who is verbally aggressive.
- Assist with the patient who is physically aggressive.
- Assist with the application of appropriate restraints.
- Assist with placing the patient in seclusion.

CRISIS INTERVENTION

DEFINITION

CRISIS INTERVENTION: A form of therapy aimed at immediate intervention into an acute episode or crisis that the individual is unable to cope with alone.

Profile of a Crisis Intervention

A. The individual is typically in a state of equilibrium (homeostatic balance).

1. Equilibrium is maintained by behavioral patterns that govern interchange between the individual and the environment.

2. The individual uses learned coping techniques to deal with simple problems that arise.

B. A crisis situation develops when a problem (triggering event) becomes too complex to be handled by previously learned coping techniques.

1. Mental functioning may become grossly disorganized.

2. The individual more readily accepts intervention in circumstances of inability to resolve crisis. The patient may be left without any other alternatives.

3. If the intervention occurs at this critical point, then the probability for resolving the problem is positive.

C. Factors that may promote a crisis.

1. Threat to one's sense of security.

   a. Situational crisis: May include an actual or potential loss of job, friend, or mate.

   b. Developmental crisis: May include any change in role as occurs with marriage or a birth.

   c. The simultaneous existence of two or more severe problems. For instance, bankruptcy, divorce and foreclosure on home all at the same time.

2. Typically, the onset of disorganization begins within 2 weeks after factors have evolved.

3. The time period may be abbreviated (less than 2 weeks), or last for years, depending on the stressors, ability to cope, or any combination of other factors such as prolonged substance abuse.

Characteristics

A. A crisis is a self-limiting, acute episode that usually lasts 1 to 6 weeks.

B. A crisis is initiated by a triggering event (death, loss, etc.) resulting in the usual coping mechanisms becoming overwhelmed by the situation.

C. The crisis may evolve into a potentially dangerous situation to the person or to others; he or she may harm self or others.

D. Individual will return to a state that is better, worse, or the same as before the crisis; therefore, intervention by the skilled mental health professional is important and the need is urgent.

E. Person is totally involved — hurts all over — has or will "bottom out."

F. At this time the individual is most open for intervention; therefore, major changes can take place and the crisis can be a positive turning point for the person.

Stages of Crisis Development

A. Initial perception and comprehension of scope of problem. Generally, problems do not suddenly occur, but are the products of continued stronger and stronger underlying feelings. It may take considerable time for the patient to "work through" all of the feelings in order to arrive at a central or focal issue. Once the central issue is identified, the treatment is more likely to be effective.

B. Rising tensions and anxieties that invoke the usual coping mechanisms. Remember the usual coping mechanisms ordinarily fall short in dealing with intense feelings associated with crisis formation. This is the reason intervention is necessary.

C. Consultation with the usual supportive contact persons. Usually, unless these contacts are professional, they may lack the knowledge base to respond appropriately to the current crisis stage.

D. Familiar methods of problem solving prove unsuccessful and tensions escalate. The inability to confront the situations causing the current crisis results in frustration, which results in the accumulation of increasing anxieties.

E. Seeks new problem-solving methods; if unsuccessful, the problem remains and interferes with the individual's life. Eventually, the patient or significant other will become desperate for assistance.

1. Mental functioning becomes more and more disorganized.

2. Extreme anxiety is likely to be experienced.

3. Perception is narrowed. The individual may become less and less in touch with reality.

4. Coping ability is further impaired.

5. Situation may result in self-harm or harm to others.

6. The individual is totally involved and hurts all over.

7. Hopelessness, helplessness, lack of self-esteem, and poor self-imagery predominate. These feelings and emotions represent total despair.

Assessment of Crisis

A. Determine period and level of disorganization.

1. Extent of disorganization

2. Length of time

3. Level of mental and physical functioning or dysfunctioning.

B. Evaluate precipitant event (cause).

1. The nature of the event that triggered crisis

2. The significance of the event to the individual

C. Examine the effectiveness of coping mechanisms

1. History of experiencing similar situations

2. History of coping with similar situations

3. Ask the patient, "Why do you feel that the usual methods of coping have failed you this time?"

D. Identify situational supports.

1. Significant others

2. Agencies

E. Suggest alternative coping modes.

1. New coping alternatives

2. Situational supports

Principles of Crisis Intervention

A. Goal is the return of patient to a precrisis level or higher and maintenance of functioning.

B. Intervene immediately because it is important that intervention occurs during the time of most acute need.

C. Assess the problem and keep the focus on this problem with reality-oriented therapy ("here and now" focus).

D. Set limits on behavior or contract for behavior if destruction (of self or others) is a possibility.

E. Remain with patient or have significant person available as necessary.

F. Explore coping mechanisms available to patient.

1. Assess for personality assets and strengths. Capitalize on them. Everyone has positive assets. Increasing self-esteem is done by focusing on and enhancing personal positive attributes.

2. Do not focus on weakness or pathology. Self-esteem may be lowered if you dwell on deficits in personality or negatives such as weaknesses.

3. Help explore the available situational supports.

4. Be calm, consistent, attentive, and genuine during this interview. Trust can be built on truth and sincerity.

G. Help the patient to understand the problem and to integrate the events in his/her life.

H. Determine if continuing therapy with a professional may be needed for future support.

I. Use therapeutic communication techniques.

Nursing Interventions

A. Focus on immediate problem.

B. Use a reality-oriented approach.

C. Stay with "here and now" focus.

D. Set limits, contract if life-threatening conditions (to self or others) exist.

E. Stay with patient or have significant persons available if necessary.

F. Explore available coping mechanisms.

    1. Develop asset strengths and capitalize on them.

    2. Do not focus on weakness or pathology.

    3. Help explore the available situational supports.

G. Assist the patient in clarifying the problem and help the individual understand the problem and integrate the events in his/her life.

H. When the above steps are completed, some plans for future support should be worked out by the therapist and the patient.

Selected Crises

Crises most frequently encountered:

1. Suicide

2. Homicide — drive by shootings, etc.

3. Accidental death

4. Kidnapping

5. Rape

6. Severe injury

7. Sexual trauma

8. Other events that cause severe stress with overt consequences either immediate or eventual

SUICIDE

DEFINITIONS

SUICIDE: The act of taking one's own life voluntarily. Attempted suicide is the plan and/or act of suicide that fails. Among teenagers, attempts of suicide or the completion of the act may trigger other teenagers to attempt or complete the act, especially those who are suicide prone. To the teenager, suicide may be viewed as the final act of liberation from parental rule or an oppressive society. Whatever the perception, the silent cry for attention and the need for intervention should be heard and implemented by the alert individual. Generally speaking, persons who are contemplating suicide give strong indications that they are committed to self-destruction. The obsession — the thinking of the act evolves into the compulsion — the doing of the act. Anyone who has the need to escape from their situation is a candidate for intervention.

SUICIDAL IDEATION: The thinking of the act and its effects on significant others. This is the beginning of the plan.

SUICIDAL GESTURE: The beginning of the execution of the plan. It is the first evidence that the plan may work unless appropriate intervention occurs. "I will not be needing this anymore." "This is my favorite (object) you can have it." "I have donated all my money to my favorite charity." If there is consistency in this "plan" to give everything away, you will need to go for the underlying feeling.

• SUICIDE ATTEMPT: The act to earnestly show that a plan exists and that it can be executed. This behavior is a cry (or scream) for help!! and should not be ignored. This act is usually in the form of some kinds of self-mutilation such as cutting the wrists, drawing or carvings on the body generally where they are not readily visible and can be covered with clothing. Cigarette or cigar burns on the arms or elsewhere is a self-punishment attempt. Verbalization that "I am going to kill myself" should be sufficient reason to commence immediate intervention. Self-mutilation, the bringing of blood, is in the mind of the patient, a return to reality. Seeing the blood reminds the patient that this is reality. Paradoxically, the patient rarely reports pain that would be associated with cutting.

Suicide Intervention

> Patient; I am going to kill myself.
> Nurse: Do you have a plan?
> Patient: Yes
> Nurse: Will you share your plan with me?
> Patient: Yes, I'm going use my razor blade on my throat.
> Nurse: Where is the razor blade?
> Patient: I have it in my wallet.
> Nurse: Will you give the razor blade to me?
> Patient: Let me get it for you.

This is the suicide prevention technique that I have used many times. The first goal *is* to relieve the patient from the stress of the presence of the dangerous object and provide a safe place. The second goal is to contract with the patient to prevent further *unnoticed* attempts to commit suicide. The third goal is to "process," that is, to allow the patient to verbalize any pent up feelings that could lead to an "impulse" suicide. Contracting with the patient does not guarantee that he/she will not commit suicide, but it increases the odds that it will not happen.

Indicators of Suicidal Activity (Lethality)

If any of the following are identified during any contact with your patient, *notify the RN or MD immediately and monitor patient activity very closely!*

- If a patient regrets that a suicide plan (attempt) has failed.
- Anger that may be internalized against self or externalized in the form of overt hostility resulting in aggressive behavior. Increased chemical dependency (abuse). Use of chemicals to overcome the pain (stressors) of either internal or external factors that will provide an escape from reality.
- Denial of need for a way out, or presumption that suicide is the way out.
- Depression as evidenced by withdrawal or seclusive, isolation, inability to concentrate, failing grades, sleep disturbances, feelings of helplessness, hopelessness, and loss of self esteem.
- Giving away material possessions . "I will not be needing this anymore." This is a very loud cry for help.
- Previous failed attempts at suicide, such as self-mutilating behaviors are important to observe, as these would be strong indicators that professional intervention is required.
- A depression that is beginning to lift.

A. General nursing care for suicidal patients

1. Explain to the patient and family why the precaution are necessary.
2. Communicate to others caring for the patient regarding the change in status, therefore care is consistent.
3. Use written indicators of the precautions as deemed appropriate by the facility.
4. Implement special observations as ordered by the physician, or as found in the Policy and Procedure Manual.
5. Conduct a search of the patient's room (with permission) for dangerous materials or objects.
6. Observe and record nutritional and liquid intakes.
7. Therapeutic assignments (passes) should not be honored during the time the patient is on suicidal precautions.
8. Be a good therapeutic listener. You may find out the underlying cause of the behavior.
9. Give the patient time to discuss his/her "feelings."

B. Suicidal (lethality) patients are generally divided into three categories: at high risk, at moderate risk, and low risk.

1. High-risk patients are those who are preoccupied with ideas of suicide or self-harm and have a specific plan to kill themselves. These are actively suicidal and must be closely supervised. Examples:

    a. Verbalizing clear intent to harm themselves.
    b. Not willing to make an antisuicide contract.
    c. Exhibits little or no insight into existing problems.
    d. Little or no impulse control.
    e. Recent attempt at suicide.

    f. Feelings about self-destruction are intense and unrelenting.

2. Specific nursing interventions for for high-risk patients

    a. One staff person should be assigned to the patient as long as the risk is high with every 15-minute checks, 24 hours a day.

    b. Restrict activities to the unit. Off-unit activities should be cancelled.

    c. Room search every shift for dangerous objects.

    d. Patient will be within arms length of staff at all times.

    e. Meals will be provided on the nursing unit, with utensil count. Beware: plastic can injure!

    f. If the patient is a minor, the parents or legal guardian should be informed when patient is placed on suicide precautions, kept informed of the patient's progress, and notified when the patient is removed from precautions.

3. The patient who is at moderate risk includes those patients who have some suicidal ideation but who are assessed as having a lesser degree of intent to complete the suicidal act. Example:

    a. Patient with a suicide plan

    b. Patient who is ambivalent about an antisuicide contract

    c. Patient who has some degree of impulse control

4. Nursing interventions for those patients considered at moderate risk of committing suicide includes:

    a. Patient should be within 10 feet of staff, line of sight viewing, with every 15-minute checks 24 hours a day.

    b. During sleeping hours, the patient should be placed as close to the nurses' area as possible. Regardless of the patient's location, checks are done every 15 minutes.

    c. Staff must accompany patient to bathroom.

    d. A search of the patients room should be done when placed on suicidal precautions. This is in the interest of safety of the patient. The milieu should also be free of potentially dangerous objects.

    e. Except for urgent, medically warranted procedures, the patient may not leave the unit. If a situation should arise that requires the patient to leave the unit, it must be done with direct staff supervision. This is known as psychiatric (psych) 1:1. One patient, one staff where the staff is directly observing patient behavior at all times.

    f. The use of sharp objects is forbidden for the active suicidal patient. If sharp objects, such as electric razors, mirrors, or scissors, are to be used, they must be under direct staff supervision.Suicidal patients should never use a conventional blade razor.

5. The patient at low risk for suicide are those patients who are having suicide ideation. Examples:

      a. No active or current plan, but may have vague suicidal ideation.

      b. Willing to enter into an antisuicide contract.

      c. Exhibits minimal self-destructive behavior and is able to control most impulses.

    6. Nursing interventions of the low risk suicidal patient.

      a. Checks every 15 minutes.

      b. Frequent therapeutic verbal contact.

      c. May attend off-unit activities with 1:1 (psych).

      d. Sharp objects may be used with direct visual supervision.

    7. Patients who are low risk for suicide may suddenly become at moderate risk, or for that matter, at high risk. Only cautious, continuous monitoring will detect these subtle thought and behavioral changes.

VIOLENT BEHAVIOR

Homicide

A. Homicide is the intentional taking (killing) of another life.

B. Behaviors that require monitoring by staff.

    1. Anger toward self or another.

    2. The other person may become target of aggression.

    3. Rage is generally the mental state of emotions prior to the commiting of the homicidal act. Rage is a greatly agitated state of anger.

    4. Suspiciousness directed at a specific target (person).

    5. An underlying feeling that evolves from "I do not like (person's name)————" to feelings of "if I do not do something about (person's name)————, they will do me great damage (physical, mental, financial, emotional etc.)." "I will kill (person's name)———— to stop my mental pain."

    6. Depression that impairs the ability to reason.

    7. Sleep disturbances, hyperalertness, loss of friends, and eventual seclusion or isolation.

    8. Homicide is linked, in many cases, to excessive use or abuse of mind-altering substances such as alcohol or acid (LSD). The possibility of homicide may increase if drugs are added to the underlying feelings.

C. Accidental Death: The sudden and unexpected demise of an individual resulting from carelessness, unawareness, ignorance, or a combination of any of the above.

D. Expected behaviors of the grieving individual.

1. Crying is the most common release of emotions associated with death. It is an appropriate response. Intervention may be indicated if the crying state becomes prolonged or inappropriate.

2. Fear of the void created by the absence of the person who is deceased. Fear of the unknown associated with the very concept of death tends to make the one left behind reflect on their own fate and mortality.

3. The grieving person may blame him/herself as he/she reflects on how he/she could have altered the situation to have prevented the demise of the departed. Self blaming is a method of reducing stress.

4. Depression may result from continued repeated unwanted thoughts.of failed closure or open regrets. This is an example of ineffective coping.

5. Regret or remorse about life events that were not completed, issues that needed to be addressed, feelings that were unfulfilled, or questions that were left unanswered.

Rape Intervention

DEFINITION

RAPE: A sexual assault on a person that is basically an act of violence; only secondarily considered a sex act.

Characteristics

A. Rape is a humiliating and violent experience for the victim who experiences severe psychological trauma.

B. The victim needs acceptance of the rape. The victim needs to be supported, not treated as the "accused."

C. The victim's behavior might vary from hysterical crying and/or laughing to appearing very calm and controlled.

D. Possible immediate responses.

1. Crying, anxiety, hysteria, incoherence, agitation, fear, mood swings, and poor problem-solving ability

2. Beginning to cope: denial, appears calm and controlled, or withdrawn, and fearful. Begins to talk about feelings, expresses anger, makes decisions

3. Resolution: realistic acceptance, able to express feelings, and control anger

General Treatments

A. Counseling:

1. *Emotional*: Crisis counseling and call Women Against Rape or other Women Advocacy organizations.

a. Degree of emotional trauma, mild to severe

b. Presence of symptoms, tearing, bleeding etc.

     2. *Medical*: Immediate medical care; assess assault and degree of trauma

        a. Assist with a complete physical examination; use rape protocol to preserve legal evidence

        b. Carefully assess and document all physical damage: injuries signs of physical entry

     3. *Legal*: The patient should not bathe, douche, or change clothes; gather evidence according to rape protocol.

B. Nursing Interventions

     1. Provide immediate privacy for examination.

     2. A staff member of the same sex should be with the victim.

     3. Remain with the victim prior to and following the physical examination.

     4. Administer physical care.

        a. Do not allow patient to wash genital area or void before examination; these actions will remove existing evidence such as semen.

        b. Keep patient warm

        c. Prepare patient for complete physical examination to be done by physician (same sex as patient if possible)

        d. Physical examination includes:

           (1) Head to toe exam

           (2) Pap smear

           (3). Saline suspension to test for presence of sperm

           (4). Acid-phosphatase test to determine recency of the attack

        e. Physical treatment may include:

           (1) Prophylactic antibiotics

           (2) Tranquilizers

     5. Provide emotional support.

        a. Demonstrate a nonjudgmental and supportive attitude.

        b. Express warmth, support, and empathy in relating to the victim

        c. Listen to what the victim says and document all information.

        d. Encourage the victim to relate what happened, have her tell you in her own words if it appears that she would like to talk about the experience.

        e. Do not pressure the patient if she chooses not to talk; allow the victim to cope in her own way.

        f. During the interview, continue to be sensitive to the victim's feelings and degree of control. If, in relating the attack, she becomes hysterical, end the interview and continue at a later time.

     6. Post crisis follow-up

        a. Counsel patient to receive repeat test for sexually transmitted diseases in 3 weeks or sooner if symptoms appear.

    b. Assist patient to reestablish contact with significant people or support person.

    c. Refer to appropriate community resource for follow-up care.

    d. Keep accurate records, as they may be important in future legal proceedings.

A. Typical behaviors and feelings associated with rape are:

    1. Great fear both of the act itself, with a greater fear of violation, as well as fear of the physical act. Mentally, the sex act may be repeated endlessly (obsession).

    2. Inability to trust the opposite sex. Most rapists are known to the victim. Trust is the basis for a relationship, and in this case the trust was violated.

    3. High anxiety may be exhibited by hysterical crying, incoherence, and inability to deal with reality.

    4. Denial is evident at first by silence related to any questions regarding the rape. Slowly the victim begins to reveal the events that led to the rape but stops just short of the description of the event.

    5. Anger emerges once the initial traumatic event has been resolved in the victim's mind.

B. A reliable listener capable of accepting is critical at this point.

Severe Injury

DEFINITION

SEVERE INJURY: Any severe traumatic act causing substantial physical or mental damage, either short term or long term.

A. Possible behavioral responses

    1. Crying is a normal response to the damage that has occurred unless it becomes prolonged or inappropriate.

    2. Depression may result from internalization of the trauma in an attempt to deal with the effects. If the patient is unable to emerge from the depression, self-harm is possible.

    3. Fear of the unknown. What will be the lasting effects of such trauma? What will others think of me? These and similar questions will emerge related to imagery.

    4. If the injury is due to physical abuse, then passive behaviors may be evident when abuse is present. Probably because the trust in the perpetrator–victim relationship has been violated.

    5. An example of injury resulting from abuse of a child may be withdrawal from abuser, or adopting a trusting significant other. This is a critical step for the child to deal with pent up feelings and abuse issues. The child needs to be able to trust.

6. Change in body image may occur.

B. It is important to be able to recognize the above behaviors in order to intervene at the appropriate moment.

MANAGEMENT OF AGGRESSIVE BEHAVIOR

One of the most challenging experiences you may have will be the managing of aggressive behavior. Let me preface this by saying that (1) what is said to you during the encounter is not intended to be personal, and (2) invoking verbal and physical management is therapeutic. Before engaging in the management of aggressive behavior you must be trained. Your state or facility may require annual recertification. Each clinical facility decides what is the appropriate level of training in the management of aggressive behavior. You must *never* attempt an intervention beyond verbal, by yourself.

Patients are advised on admission of the possibility of the use of restraints and/or seclusion. Restraints and seclusion are two forms of behavior control for the "out of control patient". The patient may be requested to inform a member of the staff if the out-of-control behavior seems imminent. Patient compliance with this request is likely if the milieu is safe and consistent.

There are two categories of behavior that require constant monitoring in the mental health facility: (1) aggression with destruction of the milieu and 2) aggression with destruction directed at self or others in the milieu. The specific behavior expectations should be made known to the patient *before* intervening to manage the aggressive behavior.

Some examples of unacceptable behaviors are:

1. Beating on doors with any object.

2. Yelling that exceeds a previously established length of time.

3. Screaming is not acceptable.

4. Crying that exceeds a previously established length of time.

5. Cursing or directing profanities at or about anyone.

6. Rage reactions.

7. Attempted self-injury.

8. An increase (escalation) in inappropriate behavior.

This is not an all inclusive list, but is intended to give examples unacceptable behaviors.

A. Nursing Interventions — **all prevention and management of aggressive behavior is based on the least restrictive method or technique of controlling behavior.**
The first intervention is the prevention of aggressive behavior.

B. Verbal management is always the first level of intervention.

1 ."Can you tell me what is wrong?"

2. "I can see that you are very upset, can you tell me why?"

3. "Would you like to go to seclusion?"

C. Physical management of aggressive behavior (PMAB) should only be used when:

1. Verbal management has not controlled the behavior.

2. When there is imminent danger to persons or milieu.

3. A staff person who is credentialed in prevention and management of aggressive behavior. Only an appropriately credentialed staff may make the decision to intervene with physical management.

4. It is therapeutic (never punitive).

5. It is the least restrictive means of behavior control.

There are many different ways (PMAB) can be certified. This is the generic approach to this discussion.

D. Use of quiet room or time outs. The patient may recognize the need to leave the milieu to collect her/his thoughts. These quiet room time outs are time specific and require that the patient process feeling during the specified times.

E. A second technique of managing aggressive behavior is to have a "show of force."

1. Usually "silent." Telephoning between nursing units and announcing a "silent code on (name the unit).

2. Staff all appear at about the same time in the same place.

3. Patient is offered alternatives to behavior.

4. Patient may agree to modify the behavior

5. Patient will be given the alternative of going to the seclusion room on her/his own.

To this point in time, no physical restraints have been used. The acceptable procedure is to: (1) use verbal intervention and (2) inform the patient that the behavior will need to be changed. *Remember: Always use the least restrictive method for resolving the out-of-control behavior!*

Only after all least restrictive methods have been exhausted, staff should employ the "code" for protecting patient or milieu from further destruction. There will be an internal (within the facility) code similar to "code blue" to indicate the need for assistance with a patient if physical restraint will be necessary. **The use of restraints as punishment is strictly forbidden.**

E. The third technique is the physical moving of patient to a seclusion area — an emergency procedure. **This is to be done in accordance with the established policy and procedure (PMAB) of the facility.**

1. The focus of treatment in seclusion is to enable the patient to regain control of her/his behavior.

2. Anytime a patient is in seclusion, the safest method of observation is one to one (1:1), line of sight and every 15 minute checks. In some cases, State law requires that staff be in attendance, within 10 feet of the patient at all times he/she is in seclusion.

3. The patient must be told the exact behavior expected to leave seclusion.

4. A written physician order is required for seclusion. The order must contain both the date and time.

5. Each order shall be time limited and should not exceed 24 hours.

6. Standing or PRN (as needed) orders should not be used (may not be legally valid).

7. Reinstatement of seclusion requires another physician order.

8. Documentation of seclusion/restrictions should describe specific rationale and behaviors that necessitated the seclusion.

9. Patients in locked seclusion should be provided:

   a. Regularly prescribed meals and fluids served with safe utensils, and if the meal or liquids are refused or after eating, the eating tray and utensils should be removed from the seclusion area immediately for safety.

   b. Regularly prescribed medications as ordered by the physician.

   c. A bath at least once daily or more often if needed.

   d. Bathroom privileges (BRP), at least every 2 hours, or as necessary.

   e. A room of adequate size (at least 100 square feet), free of hazardous objects, adequately ventilated, and temperature controlled with adequate lighting (should have a natural source of light).

   f. Articles of clothing or other items with which the patient might injure her/himself should be removed, for example, belts, and shoe strings .

10. Upon release from seclusion, the patient should be placed on an every 15-minute observation.

F. The fourth technique, if everything else has failed and the behavior continues, is seclusion with restraints.

   1. There are a variety of restraint devices available. Here is a list of 15 of the most acceptable devices currently in general use.

      a. Anklets

      b. Arm splints

      c. Belts

      d. Camisole

      e. Chair restraint

      f. Enclosed bed

      g. Helmets

      h. Mittens

      i. Restraining net

      j. Restraint board

      k. Straight jacket

      l. Body net

      m. Transport jacket

      n. Vest

      o. Wristlets

G. **WARNING**   Anytime restraints of any kind are being therapeutically employed, it is important to:

  1. Check circulation in the restrained extremity at least every 15 minutes; if there is an alteration, notify the charge nurse.

  2. Check the condition of the underlying skin tissue for abrasions or chafing, and if found notify the charge nurse.

  3. *Be certain* that vital functions are functioning; for example, respiration may be limited by a too tight vest restraint.

  4. Check that all nerves, especially those near the surface, are not impaired. Check for numbness or tingling in extremities. If found report to the charge nurse.

  5. Ensure that muscles are periodically exercised to assure freedom from spasm(s).

  6. *For your safety*, when releasing the patient from restraints, release only ONE one limb at a time. Release one lower extremity, then one upper extremity, next the second lower extremity, and then the remaining upper extremity.

H. Here is a list of unacceptable physical (mechanical) restraints.

  1. Metal wrist or ankle cuffs

  2. Rubber bands as fastening devices

  3. Rope or cord

  4. Long ties, i.e., "leashes"

  5. Restraining sheets

  6. Padlocks or key locks

  7. Restraining a patient in a standing position to a stationary object

Alternative Treatment — Nursing Management of Patients in Seclusion and/or Restraints

These are treatment approaches that may be used for aggressive patients.

A. Seclusion for time out: place the patient in an area without reinforcement for the inappropriate behavior. This area may be other than the patient's living area, such as the bedroom, courtyard, or quiet room.

  1. Institute time out immediately following each display of the specified target behavior.

  2. Use a minimum of emotional expression and verbal interaction, other than briefly announcing why the consequence has been applied.

  3. As little as 5 to 10 minutes may be all that is necessary for the patient to regain control.

B.   Social extinction: lack of staff attention to the inappropriate (maladaptive) behavior may reduce the frequency of the patient's response.

    1.   Nursing staff must be consistent in ignoring the maladaptive behavior to increase the effectiveness of this approach.

    2.   Used only for behavior that craves attention.

C.   Socialization and recreation: offer recreational materials and structured activities to avert disruptive behavior.

D.   Verbal skills technique: use verbal interaction to reduce anxiety and help the patient gain control. Speak quietly and calmly to agitated patients and allow them to express their feelings.

E.   Preventive intervention: be aware of predictable patterns, such as verbal abuse and pacing, that signal impending aggressive behavior.

    1.   Initiate effective alternative treatments such as those listed above, to deter aggressive behavior.

    2.   Inform patients upon admission that seclusion is used at the facility and why it is used, when it is used, and how long it lasts.[1]

S U M M A R Y

The key concept to be learned in this chapter is the intervention for suicide. The second concept is the appropriate care for those patients who exhibit aggressive behavior.

Review Questions

1.   Which of the following is the least restrictive form of restraint to control inappropriate behavior?

    a.   Soft leather.
    b.   Wristlets.
    c.   Verbal.
    d.   A locked room.

2.   An attempt to commit suicide is most likely to occur:

    a.   Just prior to hospitalization.
    b.   Just after discharge from the hospital.
    c.   When the depression is at its deepest point.
    d.   When the depression begins to decrease or "lift".

3.   Most suicidal patients are medically diagnosed as having major depression. The best treatment for depression is:

---

[1]Adapted from Perspectives in Psychiatric Care Vol. 26, No. 3, 1990. Sherry Myers, RN,BSN

    a. Medication.
    b. Milieu therapy.
    c. Assisting the patient in the discovery of the feeling that causes the depression.
    d. Therapeutic communication.

4. The initial step in crisis intervention is:

    a. Collect information.
    b. Resolve the problem.
    c. Identify strengths and weaknesses.
    d. Inform a support group that a patient will be needing services.

5. A suicidal patient is admitted to a locked unit of a hospital. Since the patient is suicidal, the nurse will:

    a. Assess for level of suicide.
    b. Maintain "line of sight" at all times.
    c. Take vital signs at the time of admission.
    d. Notify the doctor that the patient is on the locked unit.

6. A patient who is just coming out of group was unable to ventilate her/his anger and rage. Within 30 minutes after leaving the group he/she escalates into uncontrollable behavior. The staff's initial attempts at verbal intervention to control the behavior have not been successful. The next least restrictive method is:

    a. Show of force.
    b. Physical take down and remove the patient to seclusion.
    c. Medicate the patient.
    d. Use physical restraints and notify the doctor.

7. A depressed patient tells staff "I do not want to get up, no one can help me, I am too sick." The most therapeutic response would be:

    a. "I will leave you alone for now, maybe you will feel like getting up later."
    b. "You sound hopeless, can you tell me what you are thinking?"
    c. "Let me take your vital signs and see if I can find out what is wrong with you".
    d. "It is time for breakfast, do I understand that you do not want to get up?"

8. Suicide precautions are ordered. The primary reason suicide precautions are ordered is to:

    a. Guarantee that a patient will not commit suicide.
    b. Confine patient activities to a quiet area of the patient unit.
    c. Monitor the patient for increasing or decreasing signs of impending suicide.
    d. Make sure that the patient is on line of sight observations at all times.

9. If a patient tells you "I would be better off dead" you should know that:

    a. Suicide is genetic.
    b. Suicides are never thought out — they just happen.
    c. Suicidal ideations may lead to suicidal gestures.
    d. The more detailed the suicide plan, the more likely it will be carried out.

10. Restraints should be:

    a. Locked with a key.

      b. Verbal.

      c. Used as a last resort.

      d. Used at the first sign of unusual behaviors.

Disorders of Affect and Personality

KEY CHAPTER OBJECTIVES

Upon completion of Chapter 5, the student should be able to satisfactorily assist with the care of patients with the following disorders:

- Unipolar Disorders
- Bipolar Disorders
  Major Depressive Episode
  Major Depressive Episode Subtypes
  Dysthymic Disorders
- Somatoform Disorders
- Dissociative Disorders
- Borderline Personality
- Multiple Personality Disorders
- Other Personality Disorders
- Conversion Reaction
- Hypochondriasis
- Paranoid Personality
- Schizoid Personality
- Histrionic Personality
- Narcissistic Personality
- Antisocial Personality
- Avoidant Personality
- Passive Aggressive (PA) Personality
- Obsessive-Compulsive Disorder
- Anxiety Disorders
- Hypochondrical form of anxiety
- Neurotic anxiety
- Anxiety Reaction
- Panic
- Phobias and Phobic Disorders
- Phobias and Phobic Disorders
- Eating Disorders
- Bulimia Nervosa
- Anorexia Nervosa

DISORDERS OF AFFECT AND PERSONALITY

Unipolar Disorders—One-Pole Disorders

DEFINITION

UNIPOLAR DISORDERS: Recurring depressive episodes (one or more) where none of the "first-degree" relatives, father, mother, brothers, and sisters have a history of mania. In unipolar disorder the disorder is depression. Since the depression recurs, the disease is cyclic, hence unipolar disorder. *See* depression.

Bipolar Disorders—Two-Pole Disorders

DEFINITION

BIPOLAR DISORDER: Bipolar disorder is cyclic, with episodes (Phase) of depression followed by episodes (Phase) of mania that repeats.

Manic–Depressive (Bipolar) Illness — Manic Phase

DEFINITION

MANIC-DEPRESSIVE ILLNESS: One manifestation of an affective disorder that involves mood swings of elation, euphoria, and grandiose behavior with or without a history of depression. Cyclothymic disorder is another category of bipolar disorder and refers to a milder form of the same illness.

Characteristics

A. Specific etiology is unknown. The disorder may be the result of a genetic predisposition to the illness or to increased levels of dopamine in the brain. Efforts are now being made to discover why lithium is therapeutic in hopes of solving the mystery of manic illness.

B. Women experience this illness slightly more frequently than men. The lifetime risk of developing this illness is 1 to 2% of the population.

C. The first manic episode usually occurs before age 30 (18 to 29) and is more common in the higher socioeconomic group. It may recur in middle or later years.

D. Mania refers to an obvious, elated, high mood that is evidenced by a high level of activity and general demeanor of cheerfulness.

Signs and Symptoms of Bipolar Disorder

Early Phase

A. The mood is one of euphoria, which can lead to grandiose behavior and delusions. The patient is clever and witty.

B. The individual overreacts to stimuli.

1. The individual may display rapid speech, with play on words and "flight of ideas." Flight of ideas is the rapid thinking where ideas fly through the brain faster than they can be verbally expressed.

2. Increased motor activity.

3. Increased (accelerated) thought processes.

C. The individual exhibits lack of judgment and decisions may be faulty, i.e., spends money foolishly, runs up charge accounts

D. The individual's thinking is directed at self gratification; imagination and unrealistic goals are in place but may change as this phase progresses.

E. The individual gives little attention to physical well-being. Appearance begins to deteriorate; the individual becomes unkempt.

1. Poor sleep habits with no apparent fatigue. Operates at high energy levels.

2. Poor nutrition.

3. Poor, or even bizarre, habits of grooming.

F. Behavior varies from delightful and playful to restless, irritable, sarcastic,and even antagonistic and combative.

G. If behavior is not controlled, the individual will become incoherent, overtly aggressive, and hostile.

H. The underlying feeling is depression, however, these patients are unconsciously denying that they are depressed.

Acute Manic Phase

A. Extreme hyperactivity.

B. Easily distracted.

C. Uninterrupted rapid flow of ideas.

D. Weight loss as the patient is to busy to eat.

E. Dehydration from inadequate fluid intake.

F. Highly irritable.

G. Patient may write to government or industrial officials, and the writings may contain inappropriate or embarrassing proposals or propositions. The delusional state is becoming apparent.

H. Appearance is increasingly disheveled.

I.   Mood becomes euphoric, then exalted, then frantic.

J.   The patient may begin the unintentional destruction of items.

K.   The patient may become bossy and highly verbal.

L.   Delusions of grandeur may appear.

Nursing Interventions

A. Maintain safe environment (milieu).

1. Reduce external stimuli such as noise, people, and motion as much as possible.

2. Eliminate patient's participation in competitive activities.

3. Redirect patient's energy into brief and appropriate activities. (The patient has a reduced attention span.)

4. Be consistent in responses to the patient.

B.   Establish one-to-one relationship.

1. Maintain a calm attitude that reflects concern.

2. Maintain an accepting and nonjudgmental attitude.

3. Create conditions favorable to the development of mutual trust.

4. Avoid entering into the patient's playful, joking activity if it appears to be a manic reaction.

5. Allow the patient to verbalize his/her feelings, especially hostility.

6. Don't "buy into" the delusional system. This can be easier than you think. These patients will have you believing their delusion is real. Beware.

C. Set realistic limits on behavior.

1. Set limits to behavior to provide for a sense of security.

2. Restrain from destructive behavior directed at the milieu. Rarely is the destructive behavior directed toward self.

D. Give attention to physical needs.

1. Provide a diet that is high in calories, vitamins, and fluids. Finger foods should be in constant supply for this accelerated behavior. The key here is to replace the energy that is being used up during hyper, near frantic activities.

2. Ensure adequate rest and sleep.

3. Protect the patient from inadvertent self-harm.

Major Depressive Episode

DEFINITION

MAJOR DEPRESSIVE EPISODE: A unipolar condition in which the feeling state of the individual is abnormal and manifests itself by a complex of symptoms. The symptoms may be mild and only slightly debilitating, or totally debilitating, severe, intense, and of long duration.

Characteristics

A. The most common of all psychiatric illnesses, depression is a symptom experienced by approximately 15 of every 100 adults in our society.

B. One cause is now thought to involve a genetic link; other possible causes are personality traits such as low self-esteem, neurochemical imbalances, and environmental factors.

C. Most acute depressive episodes are self-limiting and last from a few weeks (with treatment) to a few months.

D. More than half of those persons who experience a first episode go on to suffer a recurrence.

E. About 20 to 25% never return to their previous state of mental health.

F. The depressive episode's onset may occur gradually as a result of a significant life event, such as a loss or threat a to life by an overwhelming disease process.

G. The depressed person may begin working longer hours with less being accomplished.

H. He/she may experience a loss of interest in family, school, peers, etc.

I. The affect is sad, he/she may cry or verbalize discouragement, and he/she feels hopeless and helpless.

J. There may be disturbances in sleep patterns.

K. The patient may not have adequate nutritional intake, and he/she may lose weight.

L. Speech becomes slow as thought processes slow down due to overwhelming intense feelings.

M. The patient may become fixated about her/his worthlessness, the magnitude of her/his sin, and the need for self-punishment.

   1. Aggression is directed inward—toward the self.

   2. If a patient's guilt or hopelessness is denied by significant others, agitation and extreme discomfort may increase.

N. Suicide is most likely to occur after the patient has reached the bottom of the cycle and as the depression first begins to lift. Observe closely!

Assessment

A. The distinguishing quality of mood is depression; the affect is one of sadness or gloom.

B. Behavior is slowed down with purposeful movement diminishing as the depression deepens.

C. Personal appearance is neglected.

D. Thought processes are slowed down until there is a lack or inability to think.

E. Attitudes are pessimistic and self-denigrating, and focus on the problems and uselessness of life. The individual lacks inner resources and strength to cope effectively.

F. Physical symptoms may reflect a preoccupation with body and health. Weight loss, insomnia, and general malaise are typical physical features.

G. Social interaction is reduced and inappropriate. The depressed patient feels isolated but cannot resolve that condition because he/she cannot contribute to a relationship.

H. An outcome of depression may be suicide (refer to section on suicide).

Interventions

A. The nurse may have to support activities of daily living (ADL) by directing, redirecting, or assisting.

B. Listen very carefully to the patient. You are listening for changes in the level of depression as noted above. *Remember, when depression bottoms out and the depression begins to lift, the danger for suicide increases dramatically.*

C. Ensure that the patient has sufficient and adequate nutritional and fluid intake.

D. *Always* reflect a positive, nonthreatening, nonjudgmental attitude when you are engaged in conversation with the patient. *Do not* give false hopes, but reflect positive reality.

E. Always remain calm and consistent when dealing with the depressed patient.

F. Be sure that the patient is in a safe milieu!

Major Depressive Episode Subtypes

A. Depression with melancholia.

DEFINITION

MELANCHOLIA: Melancholia[1] is a morbid mental state characterized by profound painful dejection, total loss of interest in the outside world.

1. Predisposing factors appear to be dissatisfaction with accomplishments in life and loss of pleasure in the usual activities.

2. Emphasis is on the vegetative signs and variation in mood (often called involuntary melancholia).

3. Common symptoms that accompany this disorder are a general depressed mood that is worse in the morning, psychomotor retardation, or agitation and anorexia that may result in weight loss.

B. Depression with psychotic symptoms

1. This subtype of depression is accompanied by an inability to test reality: delusion, hallucination, and confusion.

a. The patient may also have severe impairment of personal and social functioning.

b. The patient may be severely withdrawn.

---

[1] DSM-III-R, p. 346.

2. Approximately 10% of those depressed have psychotic symptoms.

3. Psychotic depressions are considered to be biologically based.

Dysthymic Disorder (Depressive Neurosis)

A. Symptoms of depression fluctuate and are less severe than with the major depressive disorder.

1. Mild symptoms are present for at least 2 years.

2. Depression may be episodic or constant.

B. Psychosis is not present.

C. Several of the following symptoms are usually present with this diagnosis:

1. Low energy level

2. Loss of interest in pleasurable activities

3. Pessimistic attitude toward the future; thoughts of suicide

4. Tearful, crying demeanor

5. Feelings of low self-esteem

6. Decreased ability to concentrate

Nursing Interventions

A. Provide safe environment to protect patient from self-destruction.

B. Observe closely at all times, especially when the depression is lifting.

C. Establish supportive relationship, letting the patient know you are concerned for his/her welfare.

D. Encourage expression of feeling, especially anger.

E. Determine the patient's capacity to entertain suicide ideas.

1. Ask questions such as, "Are you thinking of suicide?" "Did you think you might do something about it?" "Have you taken steps to prepare?" "What are they?"

2. It is important to recognize a continued desire to commit suicide.

F. Focus on strengths and successful experiences that can enhance self-esteem.

G. Follow a structured schedule and involve the patient in activities with others.

H. Help structure a plan for coping when the patient next experiences ideas of suicide.

I. Help the patient plan for continued professional support after discharge.

Somatoform Disorders

DEFINITION

SOMATOFORM DISORDERS: Also called psychosomatic disorders, they are manifested cal diseases, but that cannot be explained by physical findings and may involve any organ system, and the etiologies are in part related to emotional factors.

Characteristics

A. An individual must adapt and adjust to stresses of life.
  1. The way a person adapts depends on individual characteristics and the extent of inner stability.
  2. Emotional stress may exacerbate or precipitate an illness.
B. Psychosomatic stress or anxiety is an important factor in symptom formation.
  1. If stress or anxiety cannot be expressed through verbalization, it finds expression through particular organ symptoms.
  2. The exact relationship between stress and illness is unknown.
  3. It is thought that somatic symptoms occur in individuals who have never had to resolve dependent–independent struggles of childhood; dependent needs are not met.
  4. Illness provides a focus for the individual away from the original anxiety; it provides a secondary gain, sympathy and attention from others.
C. Structural changes in body systems may occur and pose a life-threatening situation.
  1. The individual is not faking illness; it is real and requires direct medical attention.
  2. Correcting the physical illness may not alter the underlying cause of anxiety.
D. Psychosomatic illness provides the individual with coping mechanisms.
  1. It is a way to handle anxiety and stress.
  2. It is a method used to gain socially acceptable attention.
  3. It may be a rationalization for failures.
  4. It may be a means of adjusting to dependency needs. The patient may need to depend on others and finds a healthy mechanism by using illness.
  5. The illness may be a way to manage anger and aggression.
  6. It may afford a way to punish self and others.
E. Types of adjustive techniques:
  1. Repression
  2. Denial
  3. Projection
  4. Conversion
F. A psychosomatic disorder may involve any body system.
  1. Gastrointestinal system
    a. Peptic ulcer

        b. Colic

        c. Ulcerative colitis

2. Cardiovascular system

        a. Hypertension

        b. Tachycardia

        c. Migraine headaches

3. Respiratory system

        a. Asthma

        b. Hay fever

        c. Hiccough

4. Skin (most expressive organ of emotion)

        a. Blushing

        b. Flushing, perspiring

        c. Dermatitis

5. Nervous system

        a. Chronic general fatigue

        b. Exhaustion

6. Endocrine

        a. Dysmenorrhea

        b. Hyperthyroidism

7. Musculoskeletal system

        a. Cramps

        b. Rheumatoid arthritis

8. Associated disorders may be

        a. Diabetes mellitus

        b. Obesity

        c. Sexual dysfunctions

        d. Hyperemesis gravidarum

        e. Accident proneness

Nursing Interventions

A. Observe closely and assess the patient's condition.

    1. Collect data about the physical illness, psychosocial adjustment, life situations, natural stresses, strengths, etc.

    2. Report the kinds of things that aggravate or release the symptom.

B. Attend to the whole person, physically and emotionally.

C. Reduce the demands on the patient.

D. Develop the nurse–patient relationship.

1. Respect the patient and acknowledge his/her problems.

2. Assist the patient to express his/her feelings.

3. Help the patient to release anxiety and explore new coping mechanisms.

4. Allow the patient to meet dependency needs.

5. Allow the patient to feel in control of his/her life.

E. Encourage the patient to work through problems and to learn new techniques of responding to stress.

F. Provide a safe and nonthreatening environment.

1. Balance therapy and recreation.

2. Decrease distracting stimuli.

3. Provide activities that can redirect, refocus, or help to alleviate the patient's physical symptoms.

Dissociative Disorders

DEFINITION

DISSOCIATIVE DISORDERS: A grouping or clustering of personality features that have been separated from the main personality. This cluster represents an entire personality, many times totally separate from the original personality.

In some cases, double, triple and even multiple separate personalities may be seen.

Multiple Personality Disorders

Characteristics

The dominant personality may be one of any of the separate personalities, depending on the patients psychological needs at that moment. When the personality switches (dissociates), it is a total dissociation. More precisely, the new dominate personality may have no knowledge of any of the other dissociated personalities. Each of the dissociated personalities have a complete reality, memory, identity, and conscious knowledge of that particular total self.

Etiology

Multiple Personality Disorder is the result of multiple events of unescapable trauma. MPD is linked to Post Traumatic Stress Disorder and dissociative disorders. The most likely persons to be Multiple Personality Disorders are those persons who were or are victims of:

a. War

b. Ritual abuse

  c. Satanic cults

  d. Rape

  e. Sexual abuse

The trauma of the event(s) is so intense, the psyche attempts to seal them in a separate place. Eventually dissociation occurs and the first multiple emerges generally following by others. More multiple (alters) may emerge and the emotional pain is avoided by splitting these painful experiences away.

The dissociated personalities ranges from intense good (superego) characteristics to intense murderous or evil (id) characteristics. Dissociation may be instantaneous (seconds to minutes) or occur over a prolonged period of time (hours to days). The disorder may be transient or chronic. Switching is the almost instantaneous change of personalities. You are never sure which personality you are dealing with, therefore, always assess for current personality identity. There will be at least two personalities that will take full control of the person's behavior. With multiple personalities there may be 10 to 30 or more, separate and complete personalities. The goal of treatment is to fuse the alters and return control to the host.

Interventions

A. Maintain a therapeutic relationship by:

  1. Remaining calm.

  2. Be matter of fact and firm.

  3. Avoid "buying in" to the current personality.

  4. Remember, no matter which personality you are confronted with, be therapeutic.

B. Be familiar with and participate in the treatment plan as established by the team.

  1. Maintain a safe and therapeutic milieu.

  2. Avoid exposing the patient to anxiety.

  3. Listen carefully for verbalization of pending changes in the personality.

  4. Involve the patient in modalities such as activity therapy, recreation therapy, and similar activities.

  5. Reduce self-serving behaviors. That is, divert inward thinking from the self into "here and now" reality.

  6. Group therapy is appropriate for multiple personality disorders.

Borderline Personality

Definition

BORDERLINE PERSONALITY: A disorder that may have a pattern of instability of self-image, interpersonal relationships, moods, that may begin in early adulthood and present in a variety of contexts.[2]

---

[2]DSM-III-R, p. 346

Assessment

A. Assessment will include:

1. Consistently unstable effect

    a. Marked shifts in mood and attitude toward reality

    b   Feelings of blankness or emptiness

    c. Lack of empathy and shows few feelings except for anger, anxiety, and loneliness

    d. Serious lack of control of anger, frequently complains of boredom

2. Consistently unstable and unpredictable behavior

    a. Some degree of self-destructive behavior

    b. Very little or poor impulse control

    c. Although emotionally labile, the patient may lapse into periods of psychoses.

        1) May have disturbances in consciousness.

        2) Reality may be distorted.

        3) May use confabulation to her/his advantage. Confabulation is the filling in of sentences (thoughts) with ideas that flow within the context of the dialogue and that are self-serving, i.e., make the story go the way you want it to go.

    d. Experiences difficulties with school, work, relationships, and home life.

    e. Lack of common sense.

    f. Lack of ability to gain enjoyment from life.

    g. The patient may return to a former state of dependency and does so by regression.

    h. The patient may be highly manipulative.

    i. One defense used by the patient is staff "splitting". Splitting is a manipulation technique that, if successful, permits the patient to control or influence behaviors of staff or others. The split is accomplished by convincing staff members that the other staff members are exhibiting unacceptable behavior or miscommunicating to other member of the staff. The result is that staff members cannot agree on what is the most appropriate course of action.

3. Unstable social relationships

    a. Because of behaviors, the patient has a great difficulty in forming lasting relationships.

    b. The patient blames others for his/her failures.

    c. Unable or unwilling to accept responsibilities for his/her actions or behaviors.

    d. The patient is convinced (deluded) that he/she is special and deserves special attention and extraordinary consideration.

      e. The patient is unable to interpret messages correctly and responds inappropriately.

      f. Manipulation causes others to become frustrated and angry.

      g. There is a distorted perception that persons that are manipulated are good and that those who cannot be manipulated are bad.

   4. Unstable self-image.

      a. Tend to be self-destructive.

      b. Intolerant of being alone.

B. Intervention depends on the behavior.

   1. Manipulation

      a. Recognize it, treat manipulative efforts, be objective and reflect reality to the patient.

      b. Promote patient participation in the setting of realistic goals for behavior, and establishing appropriate consequences if goals are not attained within the time frame.

      c. Set firm limits on behavior.

      d. Be consistent in your interactions with the patient.

      e. Accept no gifts from patient.

      f. Be matter of fact.

      g. Do not respond to manipulation.

      h. Give patient positive feedback for appropriate behavior.

   2. Poor impulse control.

      a. Provide reality treatment such as a therapeutic description: "I see you doing ————" (whatever the behavior is).

      b. Establish realistic limits or goals.

      c. With other members of the treatment team, set in place consequences if goals or limits are not met.

      d. Encourage the patient to attend the appropriate support group: Narcotics Anonymous (NA), Overeaters Anonymous (OA), etc.

      e. Be firm and matter of fact.

      f. Serve as a role model for the patient.

      g. Provide a safe, consistent milieu.

Other Personality Disorders

Obsessive-Compulsive Disorders

A. Obsessive (the thought)–compulsive (the doing); if both coexist; then it is the thinking and the doing. Anxiety is associated with the persistence of undesired ideas or impulses; repetitive ritualistic actions alleviated anxiety.

1. Obsessive refers to repetitive thoughts that the patient is not able to control.
2. Compulsive refers to repetitive physical act(s) that the patient is not able to stop (symbolic).
3. To stop the repetitive act would result in extreme anxiety. The behavior or thought is the method to control the environment that relieves anxiety.
4. Treatment includes group and individual psychotherapy.
5. These patients exhibit the following attributes:
   a. Rigid in routine and fastidious in the exact performance of the compulsion.
   b. Overly conscientious and overly inhibited.
   c. Perfectionist, especially interested in trivial details, and insists on doing in their own way.
   d. High degree of organization to carry out the compulsion.

Nursing Interventions

A. Avoid punishment or criticism of the compulsive repeating of acts.

B. Provide climate of acceptance and understanding.

C. Orient nursing care around patient's need to perform compulsive acts or rituals.

D. Provide for the patient's physical needs.

E. Monitor closely to be sure that the compulsions (acts) do not harm in any way the patient.

Conversion Reaction

DEFINITION

CONVERSION REACTION: Anxiety that results from an unconscious conflict and is converted into physical symptoms for which there is no organic explanation.

Nursing Interventions

A. Understand that the patient's lack of concern or indifferent attitude is a symptom of the illness.

B. Recognize that illness is frequently used for primary gains, i.e., solving conflict by not solving it and removing the source of stress. Illness used as secondary gain provides the patient with sympathy and attention to physical handicap.

C. Do not confront the patient with his/her illness.

D. Divert the patient's attention from symptoms. Do not respond to patient's secondary gains.

E. Reduce pressure or demands on the patient.

F. Create a positive relationship.

G. Use a matter-of-fact approach.

H. Provide the patient with recreational and socializing activities.

I. Teach the necessities of daily living and give assistance as needed, i.e., if patient is blind, help and show how to feed self.

Hypochondriasis

DEFINITION

HYPOCHONDRIASIS: Severe, morbid preoccupation with one's own body; abnormal anxiety about one's own health.

Nursing Interventions

A. Accept the patient and his or her complaints.

B. Provide diversional activities at which the patient can succeed.

C. Use a friendly, supportive approach.

D. Provide for the patient's physical needs.

E. Assist the patient to refocus.

Paranoid Personality

DEFINITION

PARANOID PERSONALITY: One that has a perverse and continuous tendency to believe that actions of other people are deliberately demeaning or threatening.

Assessment

A. Unwarranted and profound suspicions and mistrust.

B. Hypersensitive to the actions of others.

C. May greatly exaggerate difficulties.

D. Unable to relax, someone is planning a demeaning or threatening activity.

E. Cold and unemotional.

F. Jealous and envious. Sometimes the jealousy is pathologic. If pathologic, then great anxiety may emerge.

G. The most seriously ill paranoids are those who attribute their thoughts to powerful sources, such as God or Satan. Paranoid thinkers have the potential to engage in life threatening-behaviors.

Nursing Interventions

A. Be consistent.

B. Provide a milieu that is free of unfounded messages. Avoid overheard conversations. No free-floating conversation if the patient is near.

C. Listen to the patient.

D. Go for the underlying feelings.

E. Try to ascertain whether there is a self-destructive or homicidal behavior in progress.

Schizoid Personality

DEFINITION

SCHIZOID PERSONALITY: A personality disorder in which the patient is grossly indifferent to social relationships and has a limited range of emotional experiences and expressions.

Assessment

A. Inability to express aggression.

B. Indifferent to other persons.

C. Social relations are severely restricted.

D. Often they are fearful of other people; these patients are often found in slums or skid-row sections of a city.

E. They have a tendency to daydream.

F. They tend to withdraw from reality.

G. They tend to be very sensitive and lonely.

Nursing Interventions

A. Directed at resocialization.

B. Include in unit activities.

C. Strongly praise for positive interaction.

D. Nursing care includes care of the withdrawn patient.

Histrionic Personality

DEFINITION

HISTRIONIC PERSONALITY (HYSTERICAL): A personality type that seeks excessive attention and is emotionally immature.

Assessment

A. Egotistical, self-centered.

B. "Keeps stirring the pot" to maintain excessive attention and self-gratification.

C. Reactions to ordinary events are major dramatic acts and overreacts.

D. Constantly attention seeking.

E. Tends to be controlling, especially in relationships with the opposite sex.

F. Creative and imaginative, often preferring fantasy to reality, especially if fantasy provides attention.

G. Prone to irrational outbursts.

Nursing Interventions

A. These patients need reality therapy.

B. Be consistent and accepting.

C. Do not buy into the attention seeking.

D. Be therapeutic.

Narcissistic Personality

DEFINITION

NARCISSISTIC PERSONALITY: A personality type who has a grandiose sense of self-importance.

Assessment

A. Patients consider themselves very special.

B. Self-importance alternates with special unworthiness.

C. Fantasies of unlimited success.

D. Chronic envy of those persons who they view as more successful than themselves.

E. Need constant external approval.

F. Unable to recognize how others feel.

Nursing interventions

A. Reality therapy.

B. Goal will be to diminish the amount of attention that is needed.

C. Promote introspection to contact the underlying feelings.

D. Be matter of fact.

Antisocial Personality

DEFINITION

ANTISOCIAL PERSONALITY: Formerly known as sociopathic, it is the personality of individuals who exhibit patterns of irresponsible and antisocial behaviors.

Assessment

A. Lying, stealing, cheating, truancy, vandalism, starting fights and physical cruelty are hallmarks of the antisocial patient.

B. Charming, well-liked and friendly.

C. Seeks instant gratification.

D. Very impulsive.

E. Cannot accept social norms.

F. May become irritable and aggressive.

G. Violates the rights of others without any hesitation.

Nursing Interventions

A. Goal is to reverse impulsiveness.

B. Delay gratification.

C. Instill socially acceptable values.

Avoidant Personality

DEFINITION

AVOIDANT PERSONALITY: A personality type with a preoccupation of feelings of social discomfort, fear of negative evaluation, and timidity.

Assessment

A. Preoccupied with what others think of them.

B. Easily hurt, even with minimum criticism.

C. Low self-esteem.

D. Generally socially withdrawn.

Nursing Interventions

A. Reestablishing social contacts is the long-term goal.

B. Must learn to accept criticism as constructive.

C. May be directed at overcoming depression, anxiety, and/or anger.

Passive Aggressive Personality

DEFINITION

PASSIVE AGGRESSIVE PERSONALITY: The type of individual with a passive resistance to demands for adequate social and/or occupational performance. The patient is passively expressing covert aggression.

Assessment

A. Passive attributes:

1. Sullen

2. Procrastinate

3. Inefficient

4. Forgetful

5. Dawdling

B. Covert aggressive attributes:

1. Obstructionist.

2. Irritable.

3. Has temper tantrums.

4. Has destructive feelings and behaviors.

5. Openly hostile, competitive, ambitious "chip on the shoulder."

6. Speech is biting (terse) and argumentative.

7. Harbor hate and resentment for those who would increase their level of functioning.

Nursing Interventions

A. Assess for the underlying feelings associated with the behavior.

B. Reality of the necessity of completion of work.

C. Behavior modification as a treatment.

Anxiety Disorders

DEFINITION

ANXIETY DISORDER: An affective state that is subjectively experienced as a response to stress. It is experienced as a painful vague uneasiness, tension, or diffuse apprehension.

This is a mild-to-severe psychologic disorder that affects thought and feeling process. The individual suppresses and/or represses unpleasant thoughts and/or feelings to alleviate the discomfort of the resulting anxiety. The subsequent conflicts are handled by means of anxiety reaction, phobias, obsessive–compulsive reaction, dissociation, hypochondriasis, and neurasthenia.

Assessment

A. Anxiety is subjectively perceived by the conscious portion of the personality. No apparent physiologic basis for symptoms.

B. It can occur as a result of conflicts between the personality and the environment or between different aspects within the personality.

C. Threats to the ego cause anxiety. Ego protects the person's psyche by developing defenses.

D. There may be a reaction to threats of deprivation of something vital to the person, biologically or emotionally resulting in anxiety.

E. The individual may be unaware of the conflicts.

F. The degree of anxiety is in relation to its effect on the individual.

G. Disturbing anticipation of danger—

    1. From a specific object, activity, or event.

    2. To one's life, status, or security.

    3. Individual is generally unaware of his/her behavior patterns.

H. Level of anxiety is influenced by:

    1. The extent to which the self (ego) feels threatened.

    2. The extent to which behavior reduces anxiety.

I. Varying levels of anxiety are common to all individuals at one time or another. Individuals have little difficulty talking, but conversation may be vague and superficial.

J. Anxiety can be transmitted from individual to individual.

K. Realistic anxiety can be constructive.

L. Anxiety may be placed on a continuum or degrees.

    1. Absent (ataraxia)

        a. Uncommon.

        b. Apparent in the person who takes drugs.

        c. Indicator of a low level of motivation.

    2. Mild

        a. Senses are alert.

        b. Attentiveness is heightened.

        c. Indicator of low level of motivation.

    3. Moderate

        a. Selective inattention because it narrows perception.

        b. Point at which it becomes pathological depends on the individual.

        c. May be seen as behaviors that are complaining, arguing, teasing.

        d. Can convert to physical symptoms, such as headache, low back pain, nausea, or diarrhea.

    4. Severe. The individual is unable to function, rendered neutralized;.may need to be hospitalized.

M. Secondary gains from anxiety neurosis become associated problems. Individual becomes increasingly dependent as time goes on.

Neurosis

DEFINITION

NEUROSIS: A set of symptoms that evolves from the inability to adapt the behavior to the reality of the situation. Neurosis is not a reason for hospitalization as the disturbance has not progressed to a point where hospitalization would be of benefit. *See* Neurotic Anxiety below.

1. These are the fringe benefits that the patient receives from the symptoms.
2. Secondary gains reinforce neurotic behavior.
3. Common defense mechanisms include repression and projection.
4. Evidence of low self-esteem is observable.
5. No gross distortion of reality.
6. Personality is not disorganized.
7. The martyr syndrome is common.
8. The individual is highly suggestible.

Hypochondriacal Form of Anxiety

Assessment

A. The patient's preoccupation with the body and with the fear of presumed disease of various organs.
B. The patient does not reach delusional quality of psychotic depressions.
C. There is no actual losses or distortions of function as with hysterical neurosis
   1. Paralysis, blindness, with conversion neurosis
   2. Amnesia, sleepwalking with dissociative type of hysterical neurosis

Nursing Interventions

Treatment involves biofeedback, individual and group psychotherapy.

Neurotic Anxiety

Assessment

A. Disproportionate to the danger.
B. Involves repression and dissociation.
C. Behavior is relatively ineffective and is inflexible.
D. Anxiety is always present in emotional disorders.

Nursing Interventions

A. Intervene when patient is unable to cope with anxiety or is ineffective at reducing it.

B. The patient may be aware of his/her anxiety.

C. Maintain a positive attitude toward the patient.

1. Acceptance

2. Matter-of-fact approach

3. Willingness to listen and help

4. Calmness and support

D. Recognize anxiety-produced behavior.

E. Provide activities that decrease anxiety and provide an outlet for energy.

F. Establish a person-to-person relationship.

1. Allow the patient to express feelings.

2. Proceed at the patient's pace.

3. Avoid forcing the patient to express feelings.

4. Assist the patient in identifying anxiety.

5. Assist the patient in learning new ways of dealing with anxiety.

G. Provide appropriate physical environment that is:

1. Nonstimulating

2. Structured

3. Arranged to prevent physical exhaustion or self-harm

H. Administer medication as directed and, after anxiety assessment, if needed.

I. Understand and recognize own (nurse) feelings, limits, and attitudes in dealing with the anxious patient.

J. Remain with extremely anxious patient and use therapeutic communication.

K. Avoid using labels (strange, bizarre, etc.) for patient's behaviors.

L. Be alert to the specific needs of the patient as demonstrated by his/her behavior

Anxiety Reaction

A. Anxiety is diffuse (free-floating). Vague sense of dread that something terrible is going to happen. Attack may be sudden onset of panic.

B. Anxiety cannot be controlled by means of defense mechanisms.

C. Psychological symptoms are:

1. The patient is not able to concentrate on work.

2. The patient may feel depressed and guilty.

3. The patient may be harboring fears of sudden death or insanity.

4. Dreads being alone.

5. Confused.

6. Appears physically tense.

7. May be agitated and/or restless.

D. Physiological symptoms are:

   1. Tremors
   2. Dyspnea
   3. Palpitations
   4. Tachycardia
   5. Numbness of extremities
   6. Chest pains
   7. Nausea
   8. Increased or decreased appetite
   9. Increased need to empty bladder
   10. Dry mouth
   11. Increased blood supply in muscle tissue
   12. "Fight or flight"
   13. "Butterflies" in stomach, nausea, vomiting, cramps, diarrhea

E. Specific nursing approaches to the patient with anxiety disorder.

   1. Calm, serene approach with recognition of own anxiety.
   2. Nonverbal reassurance.
   3. Listen.
   4. Provide physical outlet for anxiety.
   5. Remain with patient.
   6. Decrease environmental stimuli.

      a. Extremely painful psychologically.
      b. Nursing intervention is always indicated.
      c. Anxiety drains energy.
      d. Defense mechanisms may be used to "solve" the underlying problem.
      f. Behavior becomes automatic.
      g. All senses are gravely affected.

F. Medical treatment may consist of psychotherapy and/or minor tranquilizers.

Panic

Assessment

A. Individual is overwhelmed.
B. Personality may disintegrate.
C. Condition is now pathological.
D. Anxiety cannot be tolerated very long.

   1. Individual cannot control his/her behavior.

   2. Individual feels helpless.

   3. Individual may be become temporarily psychotic.

E. Observed behavior:

   1. Ineffective thinking such as lack of insight.

   2. May appear wild and desperate, causing possible bodily harm to self and others.

F. Needs immediate intervention.

   1. Physical restraints following attempts to verbally restrain.

   2. Constant presence of attendant.

   3. Tranquilizers as ordered by physician.

   4. Nonstimulating environment.

Phobias and Phobic Disorders

DEFINITION

PHOBIAS AND PHOBIC DISORDERS: Immense, intense fear of a situation or object which the patient clearly recognizes as not really dangerous to self. A morbid fear with a morbid anxiety.[3]

A. Treatment is necessary if fear disturbs daily living

B. Treatment involves behavior therapy, psychotherapy, and major or minor tranquilizers.

C. By using the defense mechanism, displacement, anxiety is transferred from the original source to a symbolic idea or situation.

D. Phobic disorder are classified into three types.

   1. Agoraphobia

      a. Marked fear of and avoidance of being alone or in public places where escape might be difficult or help not available in case of sudden incapacitation.

      b. Increased constriction of normal activities; fear dominates the individual's life.

   2. Social phobia

      a. A persistent irrational fear and compelling desire to avoid a situation in which the individual is exposed to scrutiny by others.

      b. Fear of acting in a way that might be humiliating or embarrassing.

      c. Distress about disturbance and feelings.

   3. Simple phobia

      a. A persistent irrational fear and compelling desire to avoid an object or a situation other than agoraphobia or social.

Nursing Interventions

A. Slowly develop a trusting relationship with the patient.

---

[3] Psychiatric Dictionary, p. 467.

B. Do not force patient into feared situations.

C. Divert patient's attention from the phobia.

D. Direct patient's focus to awareness of self.

E. Encourage but do not force patient to discuss fears and feelings.

F. Support patient during program of phobic desensitization.

EATING DISORDERS

Anorexia Nervosa

DEFINITION

ANOREXIA NERVOSA: Gross disturbances in eating behavior, by refusal to maintain body weight above the minimum normal for age and height; accompanied by an intense fear of gaining weight or becoming fat; also these patients have a distorted body image; and in women amenorrhea may develop.

Assessment

A. A loss of 15% of body weight.

B. The patient may induce vomiting after meals. This is called purging.

C. May use laxatives and/or enemas on a daily or at least frequent basis.

D. The patient may use diuretics either over-the-counter or prescription.

E. The patient is likely to have bradycardia.

F. The patient may have hypotension.

G. The patient may hoard, conceal, crumble, or throw food away, if unobserved.

H. Of the anorexic patients 95% are women.

I. Death will occur if anorexia is persistent and untreated.

J. The onset may be due to overwhelming stressors.

Nursing Interventions

A. Self-image restoration is important.

B. Self-esteem is important.

C. Identification of the underlying feelings.

D. Daily weights.

E. Observe during meals and for at least 1 hour after the meals. Set time limit for meals.

F. Contract with the patient to "not purge" after meals.

G. The focus is not the intake of food, but rather it is the underlying feelings.

Bulimia Nervosa

DEFINITION

BULIMIA NERVOSA: Recurring episodes of binge eating; lack of control of overeating behavior during binge episodes; a persistent overconcern with body shape and weight. Generally, these patients have averaged two binge eating episodes a week for the last 3 months.

Assessment

A. Eating and eating binges may be planned events.

B. Food consumed often has high caloric content, is sweet, and has a texture that facilitates rapid eating.

C. Binges often occur secretly or are done in private.

D. The food is not chewed unless absolutely necessary, just swallowed.

E. The binge usually stops when:

    1. There is abdominal discomfort or pain.

    2. If sleep begins.

    3. There is social interruption of the binging.

    4. There is nothing left to vomit.

F. A depressed mood usually follows the binge purge cycle.

Nursing Interventions

See Anorexia

SUMMARY

As you review these disorders, keep in mind the key distinguishing features and consider how you would construct a nursing care plan for each using the APIE format. Write a plan of care for any five of these disorders based on your first hand experience with them.

Review Questions

1. You are interviewing a patient who is having anxiety. Anxiety is expressed through emotional feelings. Which of the following behaviors is least likely to be observed in an anxious person?

    a. Fear.

    b. Phobia.

    c. Hostility.

    d. Depression.

2. Paranoid thinking is characterized by feelings of:

   a. Anger and aggression.
   b. Suspicion and jealousy.
   c. Self-pity and self-centeredness.
   d. Simultaneous hero worship and hero hating.

3. Two outstanding features of paranoia are:

   a. Grandiosity and poverty.
   b. Poverty and persecution.
   c. Persecution and poisoning.
   d. Grandiosity and persecution.

4. A patient has been admitted to the Adult Psychiatric unit who has just been diagnosed as having peptic ulcer disease. Peptic ulcer disease may be considered a psychosomatic illness. Psychosomatic diseases are:

   a. Emotional disorders, where the etiology is unknown.
   b. Physical disease caused by physiologic dysfunction.
   c. Emotional disorders in which physical symptoms symbolize emotional conflict.
   d. Physical disorders caused by long-term emotional responses to stressors in the environment.

5. You are assigned to care for a patient who is diagnosed Manic Depressive, Manic phase. From your knowledge of manic phase, you expect to see an overactive patient. You notice that the patient is overactive and losing weight from the time of admission. Which of the following would help to meet the nutritional needs of the patient?

   a. Sit with the patient at meal times and encourage her/him to eat.
   b. Serve large quantities of high calorie foods and beverages.
   c. Make the patient sit in the dining room for 20 minutes, whether he/she eats or not.
   d. Provide the patient with nutritious snacks or finger foods during periods of hyperactivity.

6. The borderline (sociopathic) personality:

   a. Realized consequences of her/his acts but does not care.
   b. Learns from bad past experiences.
   c. Does not learn from bad past experiences or worry about consequences.
   d. Tries to forget about the past.

7. To care for a patient with obsessive-compulsive disorder who is observed performing ritualistic behaviors, the nurse should:

   a. Try to keep the ritualistic behavior at a minimum.
   b. Act out the ritual with the patient.
   c. Allow the patient to act out unharmful ritualistic behaviors.
   d. Stop the behavior by any means available.

8. A patient comes to the nurses station and tells you that he/she is having continual severe recurring thoughts about killing her/his spouse. You would recognize

that this thinking is termed:

a. Obsessive.
b. Compulsive.
c. Phobic.
d. Hallucination.

9. A person who continually washes her/his hands can be said to have which kind of thinking?

a. Hypochondriac.
b. Delusional.
c. Compulsive.
d. Obsessive.

10. When you are working with a patient who has an active eating disorder, you should:

a. Focus on the amount of food eaten by performing a calorie count at each meal.
b. Make it obvious to the patient that you are observing him/her eating.
c. Assist the patient in discovering what feelings could be the cause of the disorder.
d. Know the whereabouts of the patient for at least 2 hours after meals.

Schizophrenic Disorders

KEY CHAPTER OBJECTIVES

Upon completion of Chapter 6, the student should be able to identify satisfactorily correct answers to questions regarding the following knowledge areas:

- Schizophrenic disorders
- Types or forms of schizophrenia
- Nursing care of the schizophrenic patient

SCHIZOPHRENIC DISORDERS

DEFINITION

SCHIZOPHRENIC DISORDERS: Schizophrenia is a mental disorder that is characterized by a "splitting of the personality." Simply stated, "thought disorders caused by separating thought processes and emotions, accompanied by distortion of reality, delusions, hallucinations, fragmentation of personality and bizarre behavior"[1] that varies from patient to patient. The clinical course of the illness varies from patient to patient as the thoughts and feelings vary.

We will invest ourselves in reviewing the types or forms of schizophrenia.

Characteristics

A. Schizophrenia may be the result of many variables: genetics, individual adaptive patterns, poor family relationships, lack of ego strength, earlier traumatic experiences, or distorted perceptions.

B. Regression and repression are regarded as the primary mechanisms of schizophrenia.

C. Major maladaptive disturbances include impaired interpersonal relationships, ineffective mental and emotional processes, and disturbances in obvious behavior patterns.

D. These individuals generally demonstrate personality disorganization and coping difficulties.

I. Schizophrenic reactions may be either acute and/or chronic or chronic with acute episodes.

Assessing the Primary Disturbances

A. The patients' thoughts are confused and disorganized, therefore, the ability to communicate clearly may be limited.

B. Feelings (affect) may be expressed in an inappropriate manner.

C. Behavior may be bizarre or lack purposeful direction.

D. Close and trusting interpersonal relationships are difficult to establish with these patients.

Definitive Features

A. The four "A's."

1. Affect—feelings or subjective aspect of emotions are minimal, i.e., "flat affect," apathetic, inappropriate expression of moods, and responses.

---

[1] *Webster's New World Dictionary*, 2nd college ed., Simon and Schuster, 1982, p. 1273.

2. Associative looseness—no connection between thoughts and expressed ideas; difficulty in discerning logical from illogical thought.

3. Autistic thinking—thoughts are self-serving and focus inward, i.e., patient uses neologisms or invented words and lives in a world of fantasy.

4. Ambivalence—two equally strong feelings, such as love and hate, neutralize each other and may mentally immobilize the patient.

B. Other important features.

1. Reality testing difficulty—objective facts cannot be distinguished from wishes or imagination.

2. Delusions—fixed misinterpretation of reality. False beliefs maintained despite evidence to the contrary.

3. Hallucinations—sensory input (smell, taste, sound, touch, sight) that has no basis in the real world. One "hears" voices, "sees" visions, etc.

4. Withdrawal—behavior that signifies the patient's desire to regress into a more satisfying world of her/his own making (autism).

5. The above signs may manifest themselves in singularly or in combination.

6. Memory disturbances—disorders in sequencing of memory.

7. Perception of body image by patient may be disturbed.

8. Changes in speech and writing.

a. Word salad—uses words or phrases that have no logical meaning and not connected to thought.

b. Neologisms—made up or new word(s) that have no meaning to anyone except the inventor of the word(s).

c. Writing may be incoherent.

C. *Hallucinations are the apparent perception of an external object when no such object is present.*[2] Hallucinations are purely subjective and may involve any or all of the senses, auditory (hearing), olfactory (smell), gustatory (taste), visual (eyes) and tactile (touch).

1. Behaviors most associated with hallucinations:

a. Patient may complain of hearing voices that others do not hear.

b. Can accurately describe smells that others cannot detect.

c. May experience sensations on the skin (see or feel) that cannot be confirmed by staff.

d. May engage in conversation with themselves.

e. Behavior may be the result of "being told" to do a specific act. "They told me to _____."

f. Patient may appear fearful and/or frightened.

---

[2] *Psychiatric Dictionary*, 5th ed., Campbell, 1981, p. 272.

    g. Attention may be diverted from the present conversation to "listening" to someone else, who is unseen.

    h. May appear to be following someone or something by following it with their eyes.

    i. May use terms like, they, voices, etc.

2. Plan

    a. Be able to improve contact with reality by making fewer references to "they" and voices.

    b. To be able to interact appropriately without indications of nonreality. The hallucinations will no longer be present.

3. Interventions to relieve hallucinations.

    a. Assess frequency of hallucinations.

    b. Assess for senses that are involved in the hallucinations.

    c. Assess for any increase or decrease in intensity of the hallucinations. Sometimes the hallucinations may fade in or out, or be less or more intense.

    d. During the periods of intense hallucinations:

       1) Maintain a safe and therapeutic milieu.

       2) As much as possible, remain with the patient.

       3) Verbally, indicate your support.

       4) Let the patient know that he/she is in a safe place, and allow the patient to verbalize feelings that he/she may be having.

    e. Do not confirm or deny the hallucinations, but go for the underlying feelings. "I understand that you feel you are hearing voices, can you tell me what they are saying?" The feelings are more important than the voices.

    f. Remind the patient that "it is okay not to hear voices."

    g. Encourage the patient to let you know when he/she is experiencing hallucinations. "Will you let me know when you are hearing voices?"

    h. If the hallucinations are encouraging the patient to harm/kill herself/himself, you will need to know to provide the appropriate intervention.

    i. Do not become involved in the hallucination, in any way.

    j. When you are responding to the patient, always do so from a reality base.

    k. Initially, the hallucinations may control the patient and her/his behavior. Over a period of therapeutic interventions, you will observe that the patient may be able to control the hallucinations.

4. Outcome evaluations

    a. Have the hallucinations decreased or increased?

    b. Has the patient's fears and anxieties lessened or increased?

    c. Is the patient able to interact with others in a reality-based milieu?

    d. What mechanisms did the patient use to gain control of the hallucinations?

e. Has the patients level of functioning improved?

NURSING INTERVENTIONS

A. General approaches

1. Establish nurse–patient relationship.

   a. Develop positive and trusting relationship.

   b. Provide a safe and secure environment.

2. Stress situational reality.

   a. Help patient to reality-test and come out of fantasy world.

   b. Involve the patient in reality-oriented activities.

   c. Help the patient to find satisfaction in the external environment.

3. Accept the patient as he or she is.

   a. Do not deny the existence of the disturbed thoughts or fantasies.

   b. Do not deny the existence of the patient's sense of self by your responses.

4. Use only therapeutic communication techniques.

   a. Encourage patient to express all negative and/or positive emotions.

   b. Encourage the patient to express thoughts, fears, and problems.

   c. Match your nonverbal with your verbal communications.

   d. Communicate clearly with the patient.

B. Approaches to specific behaviors/delusions

The patient who is delusional has gone to extremes to develop a framework within which he/she can maintain feelings and emotions. Unfortunately, during the construction of this framework, erroneous information has been incorporated into the delusion, and the patient has or is experiencing a separation from reality. *Delusions are false or distorted beliefs, that are not based in fact.* Hence, the patient, believing that his/her perception is true, often relays information that is out of context, distorted, partially true, or is totally false and illogical. These delusions arise from the inability of the patient to deal with these underlying feelings and form reality.

The following are examples of the various forms that delusions may take (keep in mind that this is not an exhaustive list).

1. Delusions of persecution are false beliefs that others are out to get her/him; out to destroy her/him; plotting and planning, for example, as a set-up for destruction, discriminate, or otherwise to ridicule, or degrade. This perception is viewed by the patient to be absolutely true.

2. Delusions of grandeur are false beliefs that he/she is God; he/she is the chairperson of the board of a powerful corporation and in direct control of every subordinates activity and behavior. That he/she is another famous/infamous

person such as the Devil, Hitler etc. The key features seem to be omnipotence and total control.

3. Delusions of reference are false beliefs that whatever is being said, is being solely directed at the patient. To explain, if a speaker was delivering a speech to 100,000 people, the patient's perception would be that the entire message was directed solely at her/him, and that the rest of the audience was merely listeners, without any vested interest. Whatever is being said *only* applies to the patient.

4. Delusions of sin and guilt are false beliefs that all that has and is happening is the result of the patient's evil ways. That there can be no good because everything is based in evil deeds that arise from previous sin and the associated guilt. The patient believes that he/she has committed sin and that the guilt is overwhelming. The patient's life of sin and guilt is now responsible for everything that is happening.

5. Delusions of influence are false beliefs that external forces (unseen, unfelt, unheard, etc.) are responsible for what is occurring. Horoscopes are an example of influences that may be found in nearly anyone's life. Of course, this is because everyone is born under one sign or another.

The above examples are not inclusive. Delusional patients attempt to build into their delusions whatever will fit (sometimes from whatever you give them). Patients are generally unable to admit that the delusion is not true and they attempt to manipulate others into "buying" into the delusion(s). Patients tend to misinterpret and miscommunicate information as the information is "filtered" through their delusion; they tend to exaggerate known facts.

Goals for the delusional patient

1. There will be a decrease in delusional thinking.

2. The verbalization of specific delusions will be limited.

3. The patient will be able to verbalize possible reasons for the delusions.

4. The thought patterns will not reflect any delusional thinking, and the patient will be able to function without the delusions.

D. Interventions of patients with delusions

1. Help the patient to recognize distorted views of reality.

   a. Determine severity of delusional thinking.

   b. Assess whether or not the delusion is singular. If the delusion is plural (diffuse), try to determine the extent (grandeur, etc.).

   c. Find out the causes of the distorted thinking. For example, substance abuse may be the underlying cause of the delusion.

   d. Try to determine if there is any basis in fact for any component of the delusion.

   e. Are there any other thought processes present that might represent altered thought? For example, hallucinations.

2. Focus on the patient's strengths (assets).

3. Provide a safe, nonthreatening milieu.

4. Divert focus from delusional material to reality.

5. Provide situations that can create successful experiences for the patient.

6. *Do not* attempt to argue with the patient about the delusion since this would likely cause a concentration of the delusion. *Do not* deny the patient the delusion. Remember it is the mechanism for relieving the underlying feelings.

7. Affirm and reaffirm reality.

8. Always try to get the patient to explain the meaning of her/his communication. This technique will assist you in defining the underlying feelings. "I know that you feel that you are the King of Arabia, can you tell me about your feelings?"

9. Be a part of a staff that is consistent and therapeutic.

10. Be sure that the patient knows that trust is the basis for your interactions.

11. To the degree that your patient is safe, allow her/him to make choices and be in control of the delusions.

12. When delusions are in progress, redirect and refocus the patient into a reality-based milieu.

E. Specific nursing responses

1. Avoid confirming, denying, or feeding into the delusion.

2. Stress the reality of here and now.

3. Respond to the patient's feelings, i.e., validate his/her feelings by saying, "I sense you are afraid. Is this true?"

F. Outcome evaluations

1. Has the patient been able to accept reality and deny the delusion?

2. Is the patient able to function in reality without the delusions?

3. Have the delusions ceased?

4. What methods or techniques does the patient employ to minimize the delusions?

SCHIZOPHRENIC SUBTYPES

A. Catatonic type

1. Secondary symptoms of motor involvement are present.

a. Diminished activity results in bizarre posturing. Waxy flexibility is the positioning by other than the patient of a patient's arm, once positioned, it remains there until repositioned.

b. Overstimulation leads to agitation.

    2. Negativism: doing the opposite of what is asked.

       a. Rigidity is the simplest form of negativism.

       b. Mute behavior is another form of negativism.

B. Disorganized type

    1. Inappropriate affect: giggling or out of control or inappropriate laughter (formerly labeled hebephrenia)

    2. Disorganization of speech

    3. Regression

    4. There will be no systematized delusions.

C. Undifferentiated schizophrenia

    1. This type is characterized by a combination of symptoms, none of which is identified as a specific type of disorder.

    2. Flat affect and/or autism is usually present.

    3. Association disorders and thought disturbance, such as delusions or hallucination, are usually present.

    4. This condition may include other behavioral maladaptations.

D. Paranoid schizophrenia

    1. A type of schizophrenic reaction that is manifested by delusions, especially delusions of persecution.

    2. Characteristics

       a. The individual is extremely suspicious and withdraws from emotional contact with others.

       b. The onset is gradual and usually occurs between the ages of 30 and 40.

       c. Certain traumatic or stressful events in the individual's life may precipitate onset of paranoid reaction.

         1. Real or imaginary loss of loved one.

         2. Experiences of failure with subsequent loss of self-esteem.

       d. Individual expresses abnormal concern with health (hypochondriasis).

         1. Complains of insomnia and weakness.

         2. Complains of strange bodily sensation.

         3. Complains of other somatic disturbances.

       e. Individual may project paranoid or delusional thoughts.

         1. Feels persecuted, i.e., individual fears that people are out to harm, injure, or destroy him/her.

         2. Behaves as if in a state of grandeur.

         3. Expresses jealousy.

    3. Assessment

       a. May be extremely suspicious and mistrusts others.

b. May show hostility toward others.

c. May be having delusions of persecution or grandeur.

d. May exhibit chronic insecurity, inadequate self-concept, low self-esteem.

e. May have a chronic high anxiety level.

f. The patient may deny the delusion.

g. Hypochondriasis.

NURSING INTERVENTIONS

A. Establish a trusting relationship.

1. Be consistent and friendly despite the patient's hostility.

2. Avoid talking and laughing when the patient can see you, but not hear you.

3. If the patient is very suspicious, he/she will relate to one-to-one therapy more than to a group situation.

4. Involve the patient in the treatment plan.

5. Provide nonpunitive support, i.e., no threats, put downs or judgments.

B. Reduce anxiety associated with interpersonal interactions to reduce the paranoid schizophrenic thought process.

1. Avoid power struggles, i.e., do not argue with the patient because he/she may become increasing anxious and hostile.

2. Proceed with nursing treatment slowly because a paranoid patient is suspicious and often mistrustful. Explain fully the procedure before performing it.

3. Be consistent and honest.

C. Help patient distinguish between delusion and reality (refer to section on delusions).

1. Do not explain away imagined thoughts for they are real to the patient. Go for the underlying feeling(s).

2. Use reality-testing whenever possible.

3. Focus on reality situations in the environment.

PARANOID DISORDERS

DEFINITION

PARANOID DISORDERS: Diagnosis of paranoid disorder is made when paranoid features dominate the personality and behavior of the patient.

Characteristics

A. Paranoia is characterized by extreme suspiciousness and withdrawal from all emotional contact with others.

B. The onset is usually gradual.

C. The onset of paranoid reactions may be precipitated by certain traumatic stressful events in the patient's life.

    1. Real or imaginary loss of a love object.

    2. Experiences of failure with subsequent loss of self-esteem.

Assessment

A. Intense focus on hypochondriasis.

B. Complaints of insomnia and weakness.

C. Complaints of strange bodily sensations.

D. The more common paranoid psychosis is manifested by delusional thoughts

    1. The most common delusions are of persecution (people are out to harm, injure, or destroy them).

    2. Other delusions may center around grandeur, somatic complaints, or delusions of jealousy.

E. Suspiciousness and mistrust of others.

F. Hostility toward others.

G. Withdrawn behaviors occur when the patient's underlying feelings, such as anger, anxiety, fear, guilt, begin to overwhelm. The patient is more comfortable retreating to an emotional place of safety than to face the emotional reality. A patient may not only learn to escape by using withdraw behavior, but to control by withdrawing from reality. *Withdrawal is separation from emotional reality.*

    1. Any isolating technique

    2. Aloofness or extreme shyness

    3. Unresponsive to verbal and written communication

    4. Moodiness as indicated by body language and other nonverbal communication

    5. Regression may be the primary defense mechanism

    6. Turning inward or exhibiting introverted behavior

    7. Avoiding contact with others, especially those causing the emergence of the underlying feelings

    8. Affect may flatten, in more severe forms; delusions or hallucinations may be present

    9. Failure of interpersonal relationships

H. Goals for the withdrawn patient

    1. The patient will become more socially interactive.

2. Over a specified period of time, the patient will begin to participate in group and individual activities.

3. The patient should begin to develop or renew relationships with peers.

I. Interventions for withdrawn behavior secondary to paranoia.

1. Assist patient in developing a therapeutic relationship with you.

    a. Initiate interaction.

    b. Show sincerity for a trusting relationship by being consistent in keeping appointments, in attitudes, and in nursing practice.

    c. Be honest and direct in what you say and do.

    d. Deal with your feelings incurred by the patient's hostility or rejection.

2. Help the patient to modify self-perception.

    a. Structure situations in which the patient will succeed.

    b. Focus on the patient's assets or strengths to enhance self-esteem.

    c. Relieve the patient from making choices until he/she is able to make decisions.

3. Teach the patient how to restore social skills.

    a. Gradually increase opportunities for social contacts with staff and other patients.

    b. Increase opportunities for social contact with significant others (family) as appropriate.

4. Focus on reality situations.

    a. Use a nonthreatening, therapeutic approach.

    b. Provide a safe, nonthreatening milieu.

5. Attend to the physical needs of sleep, exercise, and physical cleanliness.

J. Suspicious and/or paranoid behavior. If a person responds to her/his environment with insecurity, mistrust, tenseness, rigidity, and secretiveness, then he/she would be considered at least a suspicious, if not a paranoid person. Suspicious/paranoid persons are usually emotionally sensitive. Paranoid states are defined as: gradually developing, systematized delusional states, without hallucinations, and exhibit emotional responses and behaviors that are consistent with the appropriate delusion(s).

K. Behaviors associated with suspicious/paranoid disorder

1. The patient may exhibit hostile, impulsive, and even destructive behavior.

2. The patient may demonstrate mistrust, with no real sense of who he/she can trust.

3. The patient may exhibit secret behaviors or self-protect in the delusion.

4. The patient may withdraw from reality.

5. Strong delusions may arise such as: "They are trying to get me, because I'm so rich."

6. If threatened, the patient may have sudden outbursts of physically abusive and aggressive behavior.

7. The delusions may dictate nutritional status such as: "I am not going to eat that, you have poisoned it."

8. The delusions of accusations or persecution are usually unfounded.

9. The patient may make vague, unrealistic statements, about "others" who are out to "get me." These statements may sound perfectly rational, but they will not pass a reality test.

10. Nearly all events will be incorporated into the "obvious" conspiracy plot against the patient.

11. The more endangered or threatened, the more withdrawn and seclusive the patient may become.

12. The persecution may lead to feelings of martyrdom.

13. The patient may overreact to any action that could in any way be perceived as rejection.

14. The patient may use projection on others to enhance the feelings of persecution.

15. The patient may feel taken advantage of and/or mistreated.

16. The patient will most likely be able to give you details of an intricate plot or series of plots related to the persecutory effort.

17. The patient will most likely be able to, either directly or indirectly, give you the names of spies or conspirators who are a part of the active plot.

18. "Do you see Phyllis over there, she is out to get me because she knows I am smarter than she is." "The poor thing has not had an original thought for years." Others' jealousy can also be built into the delusion of persecution.

19. As the delusion strengthens, reality diminishes.

20. If the paranoid patient is highly suspicious, and can name *the* person who is after him/her, then the patient should be monitored for homicidal tendencies.

21. These patients will tend to lose their sense of humor.

22. In the delusional patient, all viewpoints are strictly his/her own. Everything "feeds" into that one point of view.

23. The patient may have strong guilt feelings that underlie the delusion.

24. The patient may have mild to severe sexual maladaptive disorder.

25. The patient may have mild to severe feeling of inferiority and inadequacy.

L. Suggested goals

1. To be able to verbalize a diminishing feeling of the persecution, for example, "that they are out to get me."

2. To be able to communicate with staff and peers, in a reality-based information.

3. To improve communication, moving from the delusional state into reality, by participating in group and other scheduled activities.

M. Interventions

1. The need for continual assessment of the patient that might indicate that the suspicious/paranoid behavior is diminishing.

2. Assess for the development of homicidal tendencies.

3. Try to determine the factor(s) that initially caused the onset of suspicious/paranoid behavior.

4. Use clear, concise, simple, and matter of fact words and sentences that will preclude the building of, or inclusion in, the delusion.

5. Keep the milieu clean and clear of extraneous sounds and sights that could provoke heightening the delusion.

6. Maintain therapeutic communication at all times, by being nonthreatening and nonjudgmental.

7. Avoid engaging in power struggles, this reinforces the suspicious/paranoid feelings.

8. If there are to be changes in activities, be sure to let the patient know, in advance (see #4).

9. As much as possible or as ordered, observe the patients area or territory and avoid intruding into her/his area, unless invited.

10. Set expectations for behaviors as soon as possible, within the limits of tolerance of the patient.

11. Encourage group participation to the limits of tolerance.

12. During periods of extreme suspiciousness, provide the patient with tasks that can be done by one person.

N. Evaluation outcome

1. Is the reality base improving?

2. Is the patient able to understand the cause of suspiciousness and paranoid behavior?

3. Is there evidence that the patient is able to trust?

4. Is the patient able to recognize the onset of suspicious/paranoid behavior and counter them?

S U M M A R Y

The key concepts in Chapter 6 are for the student to be able to understand:

- Assist with the care of the paranoid patient.
- Begin to understand the underlying concepts of treatment of the suspicious/paranoid patient.

- Use the APIE criteria in the developing a plan of care for the paranoid/suspicious patient.
- Use therapeutic communication when caring for the paranoid/suspicious patient.

Review Questions

1. A patient who is about to have diagnostic testing done on the next day expresses concerns about the tests by stating "I am here to find out why I have been getting these backaches and besides I do not think there is anything wrong with me." Which of the following defense mechanisms is the patient using?

   a. Denial.
   b. Aggression.
   c. Regression.
   d. Isolation.

2. Psychotic responses are:

   a. Not as severe as neurotic ones.
   b. Involve minor defects in reality.
   c. Reflected in disturbances of total personality functioning.
   d. Evidenced by hallucinations only.

3. Which of the following symptoms would a person who is diagnosed as a paranoid schizophrenic most likely not have?

   a. Waxy flexibility.
   b. Suspiciousness.
   c. Hallucinations.
   d. Delusions of persecution.

4. The characteristics most frequently associated with schizophrenia are:

   a. Apathy, ideas of reference, and autistic thinking.
   b. Flat affect, autistic thoughts, ambivalence, and associative looseness.
   c. Ambivalence, autism, associative looseness, and ideas of reference.
   d. Confabulation, suspicious, insightful, and intuitive.

5. The symptom that characterizes paranoia in its true form is:

   a. Bizarre hallucinations.
   b. Inappropriate affect.
   c. Severe depression.
   d. Systematized delusions.

6. The primary defense mechanism used in paranoid thinking is which of the following:

   a. Projection.
   b. Compensation.
   c. Rationalization.
   d. Sublimation.

7. The manner in which questions are asked can be improved by all of the following, EXCEPT:

   a. Listening before questioning.
   b. Stating questions so that only a yes or no answer is required.
   c. Phrasing questions clearly and concisely.
   d. Asking only questions that are pertinent to the subject under discussion.

8. A nursing staff member begins a conversation with a patient. The patient says "I do not want to talk today." What would be the most therapeutic response that communicates understanding and acceptance?

   a. "You say you do not want to talk today."
   b. "I will sit here with you for a while."
   c. "There is no need for you talk today."
   d. "Why do you not want to talk today."

9. A patient has been admitted to the hospital voluntarily, at the urging of her/his physician. Lately he/she has been accusing her/his neighbors of "bugging" her/his phone and "listening in" on conversations. Yesterday he/she accused her/his neighbors of plotting to "kill" her/him. The patient does not wish to remove her/his clothes during the admission process. The staff should proceed to:

   a. Get additional staff and remove the patient's clothes.
   b. Leave the room and get the orderly to remove the clothes.
   c. Find out why the patient does not want to undress.
   d. Let the patient wear the street clothes.

10. Refer to question 9. The patient is angrily telling you about what people have been doing to her/him. Your best response would be:

    a. Say nothing.
    b. "I do not blame you for being angry, the things they are doing are terrible."
    c. "It does not really make any sense does it, that your neighbors would be doing these kinds of things."
    d. "It must be difficult for you to feel all alone and threatened like that."

Addictive (Dependency) Disorders

KEY CHAPTER OBJECTIVES

Upon completion of Chapter 7, the student should be able to identify satisfactorily correct answers to questions regarding the following knowledge areas:

- Dependency disorders
- Co-dependency disorders
- Mind-altering drugs
- Polysubstance abuse
- Contribute to the assessment by gathering data, assisting with formulating a nursing plan, providing interventions, and evaluating the outcome of the plan of care regarding:

    Polysubstance abuse

    Dependency

SUBSTANCE USE AND ABUSE

DEFINITION

SUBSTANCE ABUSE: A general term that refers to maladaptive behavior that occurs as a result of the use of drugs; the degree of social or occupational impairment is less than the impairment associated with psychologic or physiologic dependence.[1] Denial is the primary defense mechanism used to continue the addictive behavior.

Levels of Substance Abuse

A. *Psychological dependence:* Emotional dependence, desire, or compulsion to continue taking the substance or drug.

B. *Tolerance:* The gradual increase of the amount required to obtain the desired effect.

C. *Physical dependence:* Physical need for the substance manifested by appearance of withdrawal symptoms when substance is withheld.

D. *Recreational use:* A part of our culture that uses "natural" substances of plant origin such as marijuana. Beyond experimentation, this tends to combine substances together for an increasingly powerful effect.

E. *Experimentation:* A person who uses one or more substances, legal or illegal, to satisfy curiosity.

F. *Regular user:* A person who engages in a continuing abuse of substance(s) to get high on a regular and continuing basis. This person tries to lead a "normal" life and carry on "normal" activities.

G. *Binge user:* A person who uses and abuses substances in out-of-control manner for a short period of time. The user usually abstains until triggered into the next binge.

Impact of Substance Abuse on Society

A. Causes of substance abuse
   1. Misinformation primarily from peer groups. Peers will introduce the euphoria associated with alcohol, cocaine, marijuana, paint sniffing, and many other similar psychoactive substances.
   2. Economics of buying and selling of illegal substance represents *billions* of dollars. This money hunger promotes the distribution and sale of illegal substances.

---

[1]Psychiatric Dictionary, Fifth edition 1981, Campbell. page 605.

3. Escape provides mental relief from reality. Unfortunately, this escape may become an addiction.

4. The medicine cabinet mentality that has been prompted by the liberal use of commercials on television, radio, newspapers, and other mass media. The wonders of the cures, and the believing and trusting in what one has read about, has lead to relief by opening the medicine cabinet. Our children then follow the role provided them.

5. Realization that substance abuse affects everyone. Nonsubstance users tend to think "it is their problem."

6. Substance abuse either directly or indirectly contributes to the following:

   a. Accidents

   b. Illness and health problems

   c. Addiction

   d. Legal penalties

   e. Financial burdens

   f. Crime

   g. Suicide

   h. Death associated with the AIDS virus

B. Prevention

   1. Information

      a. Studying available printed information.

      b. Attending workshops and seminars.

      c. Watching features presented on television and other current sources.

      d. Being aware of information related to substance abuse.

      e. Assist with identifying special populations at risk of abuse, i.e., adolescents, and *listen* to them.

   2. Education

      a. Learn/teach decision making skills.

      b. Teach how to cope with stress.

      c. Instill problems-solving techniques.

      d. Teach interpersonal skills and especially personal communication skills.

      e. Motivate the individual to learn life skills.

   3. Communication.

      a. Communicate by role modeling reflecting positive attitudes and actions.

      b. Listen attentively and encourage the individual to express feelings and thoughts.

      c. Mutual trust and respect.

   4. Alternatives

    a. Involvement in scholastic and extracurricular activities.

    b. Redirection is a plan of a new, positive course of action.

    c. Provide ample structure of time—uncommitted time is usually when most substance abuse occurs.

    d. There should be some degree of discipline. This could be stated or written rules with accompanying rewards and consequences.

5. Intervention at the earliest possible time[2]

    a. Peer associations

    b. School counselors

    c. Professional mental health counseling

    d. Involvement in AA, Alanon, NA, etc.

    e. Counselors "on the job"

Remember: Intervention always starts with a concerned, interested person. Generally, the addict's mind and body actions may be so controlled by the abuse that the addict cannot take an active part in obtaining help.

ALCOHOLISM

DEFINITION

ALCOHOLISM: The abuse of any alcoholic substance combined with either physical or psychological addiction.

Characteristics

A. Alcohol consumption is permitted by law and supported by most people in our society as a recreational activity.

B. A fine line exists between the social drinker and the addicted or problem drinker.

C. The greatest difference between the social and addicted drinker is the degree of compulsion to drink and the ability to survive the trials of everyday living without the ingestion of alcohol.

D. Alcoholism, the third largest health problem in the United States (heart disease and cancer rank first and second), affects 10 million people.

E. Alcoholism is involved in about 30,000 deaths and 500,000 injuries (automobile accidents) every year.

F. Alcoholism decreases life span 10 to 12 years.

G. Loss to industry caused by alcoholism is estimated at $15 billion a year (affecting primarily the 35- to 55- year old age group).

---

[2]Americans for a Drug Free America, American Crisis Publishing, Inc., Austin, TX: 4–10.

H. A major U.S. social concern is the dramatic rise in teenage alcoholism (estimated to affect 3 million adolescents).

I. Dependency is psychologic: Addiction is physiologic.

J. A dependent personality that resents authority.

K. Sets high self-expectations but has a low tolerance for frustration.

L. Inclined toward pattern of failure.

M. Uses alcohol to gain a false sense of success, power, confidence, and self-worth.

N. Uses alcohol to ease suffering, reduce anxiety, and help cope with life stresses.

O. Functions with less intellectual, emotional, and social ability as need for alcohol increases.

Dynamics of Alcoholism

A. Alcoholic disease implies the consumption of alcohol to the point where it interferes with the individual's physical, emotional, and social functioning.

   1. The syndrome consists of two phases: problem drinking (habituation) and alcohol addiction.

   2. Dependence on other drugs is very common.

B. No hereditary or organic basis for alcoholism has been proven to date.

C. Alcohol blocks synaptic transmission, depresses the central nervous system (CNS), and releases inhibitions. It acts initially as a stimulant but is actually a depressant.

   1. Chronic excessive use can lead to brain damage (sedative effect on the CNS).

   2. High blood levels may cause malfunctions in cardiovascular and respiratory systems.

D. Blood level of 0.15% or more of alcohol is considered the level of intoxication.

E. Psychological effects of alcohol appear to be the gratification of oral impulses and the reduction of superego forces; abuse leads to shame and guilt, impaired ego function.

   1. Patient begins to have disturbances in ability to relate socially or function economically.

   2. "Thinking" becomes focused on ability to obtain alcohol. This is called "drug - seeking behavior."

   3. Alcoholism is, for the patient, an increasingly complex disease that is incorporated in the behavior.

   4. Denial tactics frequently used by alcoholics.

      a. "I need to unwind."

      b. "This is the only way to relieve stress."

      c. "I am getting away from it all."

      d. "I feel better—the problems go away."

    e. Patients will become uninhibited in behavior.

    f. "This loosens me up, so I can socialize."

F. Jellinek's stages of alcoholism (not always occurring in the same order).[3]

  1. Prealcoholic

    a. Occasional drinking.

    b. Constant relief drinking.

    c. Increase in alcohol tolerance.

  2. Prodromal

    a. Memory blackouts

    b. Secretive drinking

    c. Preoccupation with alcohol

    d. Guilt feeling without drinking

  3. Crucial

    a. Loss of control

    b. Rationalization of drinking

    c. Aggressive behavior

    d. Trouble with family and employer

    e. Self-pity

    f. Unreasonable resentment

    g. Neglect of food

    h. Tremors

    i. Morning drinking

  4. Chronic

    a. Prolonged intoxication

    b. Physical, mental, and moral deterioration

    c. Impaired thinking

    d. Obsession with drinking

    e. Giving constant alibis

G. Alcohol may be said to be a defense against anxiety; therefore, the patient needs to work on problems causing her/his anxiety.

H. Physiologic changes associated with alcoholism

  1. Korsakoff's syndrome

  2. Delirium tremens

  3. Chronic gastritis

---

[3]Kalman, adapted from Kalman and Waughfield, 2nd ed., 1987, Delmar: 227–228.

4. Poor nutritional intake resulting in beriberi, pellagra, cerebellar degeneration, and anemia

5. Laennec's cirrhosis and hepatitis

6. Peripheral neuropathy

7. Osteoporosis

8. Infection

9. Depresses bone marrow, and thereby decreases the production of red blood cells.

10. Scars tissues of the liver (cirrhosis) which is the organ of primary detoxification of alcohol.

11. The results of CNS depression are:

    a. Staggering gait.

    b. Falling with the inability to get up.

    c. After prolonged drinking episodes, delirium may result.

12. Caused by ingesting large volumes of alcohol.

13. Impairs ability to reason.

14. Patient becomes toxic, at least to some degree.

15. Inevitably, some tissue destruction will occur.

I. Dangers of consuming alcohol

1. Neglect of diet, which may result in serious deficiencies of vitamins and minerals.

2. "Blackouts" lasting from minutes to days.

3. Impotency or decreased libido.

4. Increasing the risk for miscarriage or premature birth.

5. Physical dangers are:

    a. Ruptured veins.

    b. Heart muscle weakens and decreases the pumping action. Hypertension may be the result.

    c. Gastritis.

    d. Inflamed pancreas may be the result of alcoholic poisoning.

    e. May permanently damage brain cells.

    f. May contribute to cancer of the esophagus.

    g. Death may result as the liver becomes more and more cirrhotic.

6. Contributes to boat and automobile accidents, and death by drowning or fire.

7. Considered by many to be the link in abusive behavior.

8. Addiction.

J. Withdrawal from alcohol includes:

1. Can be fatal.
2. Tremors of fine muscles followed by general muscular involvement.
3. Anxiety.
4. Nausea and vomiting.
5. Diaphoresis.
6. Cramps.
7. Hallucinations—called delirium tremens.
8. Mild to severe diarrhea
9. Convulsions or some form of seizure activity.
10. Coma followed by heart failure and circulatory collapse.

Nursing Interventions

A. Help reestablish the patient's healthy physical condition.
   1. Provide adequate nutrition with fluids and a high protein diet.
   2. Promote adequate rest and sleep.
   3. Observe patient for symptoms of impending delirium tremens.

B. Maintain a controlled and structured environment until the patient is able to manage her/his circumstances.
   1. Set behavior limits and confront the manipulative patient.
   2. Suggest group interaction for lonely patients.
   3. Remember that the patient needs support, firmness, and a reality-oriented approach.

C. Treatment techniques
   1. Patient must first go through detoxification—intensive care to prevent the toxic state and then the return to a nonalcoholic state.
   2. Stress need for a change in attitudes.
      a. To accept the fact that alcoholism is an illness.
      b. To accept the fact that life must be managed without the support of alcohol.
   3. Promote psychotherapy techniques of group and family therapy; establish positive nurse–patient relationship for therapy.
      a. Therapy goals.
         1) Focus on the underlying emotional problems.
         2) Offer assistance in handling anxiety.
         3) The patient can be supported in efforts to change by nonprofessional groups (AA), but change will not occur unless patient wants to be helped.
      b. Encourage rehabilitation or long-term supportive care.

  c. Continued psychotherapy on an outpatient basis.

  d. Referral to Alcoholics Anonymous

4. Medication such as Antabuse (alcohol-sensitizing drug that causes vomiting and cardiovascular symptoms if the patient consumes or even comes in contact with alcohol of any kind [after shave or perfumes] after taking the drug).

5. Referral to social or vocational rehabilitation community program.

D. Nursing approaches when working with the alcoholic patient

1. Maintain a therapeutic attitude (nonthreatening and nonjudgmental) toward the alcoholic.

2. Approach the patient with firmness and consistency.

3. Accept the individual but not his/her deviant behavior.

4. Support the patient's attempt to change life patterns.

DRUG ADDICTION

DEFINITION

DRUG ADDICTION: The dependency on drugs other than alcohol or tobacco that alter perception and/or mood.

Characteristics of Narcotic Addiction

A. The most common narcotics are heroin and morphine.

B. Emotional dependence on the drug (to alter mood) is followed by physical dependence on the drug.

C. Narcotics have a sedative effect on the CNS.

D. As tolerance level increases, need for greater amounts.

E. Addiction tends to be chronic; the rate of relapse is high.

F. Withdrawal symptoms

1. Anxiety

2. Nausea and vomiting

3. Sneezing, yawning, and watery eyes

4. Tremors and profuse perspiration

5. Stomach cramps and dehydration

6. Convulsions and coma

G. Characteristics of the narcotic addictive personality

1. Emotionally immature with feelings of inadequacy and inferiority

2. Difficulty in establishing interpersonal relationships; untruthful and insecure
3. Poor judgment and inability to tolerate frustration

Characteristics of Barbiturate Addiction

A. The most common barbiturates are Seconal and Sodium Amytal.
B. Barbiturates have a sedative effect on the CNS.
C. Danger of death from overdose.
D. Emotional dependence on the drug is followed by physical dependence on the drug.
E. Originally may have been taken to relieve pain or sleeplessness.
F. Addicts usually have emotional problems and an anxious temperament.

Characteristics of Other Common Drug Addictions

Stimulants

A. Amphetamines
   1. The most common amphetamines are Benzedrine and Dexedrine; also included are Methamphetamine.
   2. They are CNS stimulants, therefore, overuse may result in brain damage.
   3. They have the effect of producing a "high."
   4. Large doses produce a hyperactive and agitated state.
   5. They produce an emotional addiction, especially for persons who feel insecure and inadequate.
   6. They reduce appetite and awareness of bodily needs so the person's physical condition suffers.
B. Cocaine, "crack" or "rock"
   1. Subjective assessment
      a. CNS stimulant.
      b. Provides a "rush" of pleasurable sensation or heightened psychic or body energies.
      c. Produces false feelings of confidence, strength, and endurance.
      d. Accelerates the pulse, increases blood pressure, and increases respiration.
      e. Greatly enhances the libido.
      f. Impairs physical activities.
      g. Usually sniffed or used intravenously.
      h. Strong psychological dependence or tolerance may occur.

     i. Does develop a physical dependence or tolerance.

  2. Objective assessment.

    a. Extreme excitability.

    b. Dilated pupils.

    c. Vital signs are increased.

    d. Sniffles, red and/or running nose.

    e. Distorted thinking.

    f. Paranoia.

    g. Sleeplessness and/or chronic fatigue.

C. Other stimulants include Ritalin, Adipex, and Fastin .

D. Withdrawal from stimulants includes:

  1. Extreme fatigue

  2. Lethargy

  3. Anxiety

  4. Depression

Hallucinogenics, LSD, or "Acid"

A. A hallucinogenic drug that mimics hallucinations seen in psychosis.

B. Produces changes in perception and logical thought processes.

C. Not considered addictive per se, but individual may become emotionally dependent on the drug.

D. Experiences following LSD ingestion range from ecstasy to terror; the consequences are unpredictable.

E. Subjective Assessment

  1. Sense of detachment from surroundings.

  2. Numbness.

  3. Distortion of reality; may be "seeing sounds" or "hearing colors."

  4. May experience visual hallucinations. May be horrible if having "bad trip."

  5. May have extreme delusions.

  6. Effects may last 10 to 12 hours. Tolerance seems to increase with increased use.

F. Objective Assessment

  1. Eyes fixed or in blank stare.

  2. Slurred or blocked speech.

  3. Anxious, restless and/or sleeplessness.

  4. Loss of appetite, with resultant weight loss.

  5. Increased physical energy.

G. Dangers

1. Flashbacks may occur even after long periods have elapsed from the original ingestion of the substance.

2. Psychic dependence.

3. Severe mood disorders and paranoia.

4. Loss of coordination.

5. Impaired judgment that can result in accidents and accidental death.

6. Violence to such a degree that the person may become a threat to self or others.

7. Genetic changes.

8. Occasional depersonalization and/or depression, so severe that suicide is a strong possibility.

PCP (phencyclidine), "Crystal," "Elephant Tranquilizer"

A. Usually smoked with marijuana; may also be ingested or injected.

B. Reactions vary from sense of well-being to total disorientation and hallucinations.

C. Considered an extremely dangerous street drug.

D. Psychological dependence may occur.

E. Cerebral cellular destruction and atrophy may occur with even small amounts.

F. Overdoses or "bad trips" are characterized by erratic and unpredictable behavior, withdrawal, disorientation, self-mutilation, and self-destructive behaviors.

G. Overdoses are treated with sedatives, with a decrease of environmental stimuli, and with protection of the patient from the self-harm and harm of others.

H. Subjective assessment

1. Great physical strength

2. Extreme agitation

3. Hallucination

4. Confusion and loss of memory

5. Increased tolerance for physical pain

6. Disorientation to time and environment

7. Schizophrenic behavior

I. Objective assessment

1. Increased vital signs—blood pressure, temperature, pulse and respiration.

2. Perspiring to diaphoresis.

3. Speech patterns become repetitive.

4. Blank stare.

5. Incomplete verbalization due to impaired thoughts and the thinking process.

    6. Drowsy.

    7. Lack of muscular coordination.

    8. Muscle rigidity in extremities.

    9. Violent, combative behavior.

  10. Slurred speech that could be described as "thick."

  11. Eyes may be nystagmatic (involuntary eye movement).

  12. Behavior may be cyclic.

J. Dangers of PCP

    1. Highly volatile chemicals.

    2. Death by "behavioral toxicity" in that the person is so intoxicated that they engage in behavior that can result in serious injury or in some cases death. An example is diving into a swimming pool, not swimming, and consequently drowning.

    3. Misrepresenting the ingredients that are added to the basic chemicals of the PCP. PCP is easily mixed with numerous other drugs (chemicals) and the user would not be aware of this.

K. Withdrawal from hallucinogenics

    1. Depression

    2. Poor memory or memory loss

    3. Confusion

    4. Flashbacks

    5. Headaches

    6. Increased need for sleep

    7. Craving for PCP

Narcotic Analgesics

A. Opium, Morphine, Codeine, Heroin, Methadone, and Meperidine

B. Subjective assessment

    1. Short lived euphoria.

    2. Impaired motor reflexes.

    3. Reduced vision.

    4. Drowsiness followed by profound sleep.

    5. Decreased physical activity.

    6. Relief from pain.

    7. Constipation.

    8. Addicting—both psychological and physiologically.

    9. May be fatal.

  10. Sleeping patterns may change.

C. Objective assessment
 1. Constricted pupils
 2. Drooping eyelids
 3. Dry mouth
 4. Fresh injection sites
 5. Low raspy speech
 6. Poor motor coordination
 7. Depressed reflexes

D. Dangers
 1. AIDS
 2. Addiction may result in:
  a. Malnutrition
  b. Infection
  c. Inability to have disease processes cared for.
 3. Reactions to contaminants as the result of using unsterile needles and injection techniques that result(s) in:
  a. Blood poisoning.
  b. Hepatitis.
  c. Abscesses.
  d. Death due to unexpected impurities.
  e. Death from overdose.

E. Withdrawal from narcotic analgesics
 1. Watery eyes
 2. Runny nose rhinorrhea
 3. Yawning
 4. Perspiring or diaphoresis
 5. Restlessness
 6. Irritability
 7. Insomnia
 8. Loss of appetite — anorexia.
 9. Tremors
 10. Sneezing
 11. Symptoms peak about 48 to 72 hours after the last dose of the substance
 12. Stomach cramps and diarrhea
 13. Increase in heart rate and blood pressure
 14. Chills alternating with diaphoresis - hot flashes, weakness
 15. Pains in muscles and muscle spasms

Marijuana

A. The abuse potential is minimal because it produces neither tolerance nor physical dependence.

B. Produces "dreamy" state and feelings of euphoria, hilarity, and well-being.

C. Moods vary according to environmental stimuli.

D. Changes in perception of space and time seem to distort and extend.

E. High dosage may produce hallucinations, delusions, fantasies, and paranoia.

F. Assessment

1. Inability to concentrate.

2. Dulling of attention, despite the illusion of heightened insight.

3. Feelings of intoxication.

4. Rapid changes in emotions from stuporous to erratic.

5. Reduced motor skill coordination.

6. Impaired memory.

7. Altered sense of identity.

8. Distortion of time and images.

9. May reduce or cause temporary loss of fertility. If consumed during pregnancy, the newborn may be premature and have low birth weight.

10. Changes in sensory perception such as heightened sense of sight, smell, taste, touch, and hearing.

G. Objective assessment

1. Very bloodshot eyes.

2. Increased pulse rate and blood pressure.

3. Muscular tremors.

4. Euphoria.

5. Inability to focus and maintain attention.

6. Disorientation.

H. Dangers

1. Lung damage of five marijuana cigarettes is equal to 125 commercial cigarettes. Marijuana contains more carcinogens (chemicals) than commercial cigarettes.

2. Continued use causes an increase in tolerance levels, thereby requiring more and more marijuana to achieve the same "high" sensations.

I. Withdrawal from marijuana includes:

1. Insomnia

2. Anxiety

3. Restlessness

4. Irritability

  5. Mental confusion

  6. Anorexia

  7. Nausea

  8. Depression

  9. Craving for marijuana

Depressants

A. Barbiturates, benzodiazepines, and methaqualone.

B. Subjective assessment

  1. Impaired vision and perception.

  2. Impaired judgment.

  3. Inability to divide attention.

  4. Depression of the CNS.

C. Objective assessment

  1. Mild to heavy sedation.

  2. Temporary sense of well being.

  3. Depressed.

  4. Slurred speech.

  5. Reduced coordination and reflex action.

  6. May have staggered gait.

  7. Disoriented.

  8. Confused.

  9. Eyes may move spasmodically.

D. Dangers

  1. The judgment is impaired.

  2. Intensity of effects are increased when combined with alcohol.

  3. The person may become addicted.

  4. Tolerance to depressants develops rapidly. This may eventually cause death when the user tries to increase the dose for maximum effect.

  5. Frequently used by women to commit suicide.

  6. If severe depressant poisoning occurs as indicated by coma, clammy skin and a weak, rapid pulse, then death may occur without prompt medical intervention.

  7. Barbiturates play a significant role in poisoning and suicides.

E. Withdrawal from depressants may include:

  1. Anorexia

  2. Restlessness

  3. Anxiety

4. Nausea

5. Increased heart rate

6. Diaphoresis

7. Trembling uncontrollably

8. Abdominal cramps

9. Convulsion

Nursing Interventions

A. General nursing approaches and attitudes are similar to those enumerated for alcoholism.

B. Special approaches to drug addiction.

1. First step is withdrawal treatment; accomplished abruptly ("cold turkey") or gradually over a period of days.

2. The substitute drug methadone is used to reduce the physical reaction to withdrawal from opiates.

3. Extended medical and psychiatric treatment for physical and emotional deterioration must be part of convalescence.

4. Resocialization process of the patient; needs supportive treatment from professional and/or community resources.

5. Rehabilitation programs must be directed toward helping the person reenter the mainstream of society.

    a. Many organizations operated by ex-addicts offer help in rehabilitation.

    b. Therapeutic communities and group therapy programs also assist with rehabilitation.

6. Specific guidelines

    a. Provide a structured environment and set consistent, realistic, and strict limits.

    b. Identify patient's attempts to manipulate; maintain control.

    c. When patient distorts reality, affirm the situational facts.

    d. Give equal concern to patient's physical, social, and emotional needs.

CODEPENDENCY AND ADDICTIVE PERSONALITY

DEFINITION

CODEPENDENCY: To join (voluntarily or involuntarily) a relationship(s) in which all emotions are influenced, controlled, or determined by another in that same relationship. The influence, control, or determinations may lead to and extend in the relationship to *total* reliance on the other.[4]

A. Factors associated with codependent relationships may be:

1. Birth

2. Substance abuse

3. Behavior (usually unacceptable ones).

4. Must speak the same dysfunctional language, alcoholics codepend with alcoholics.

B. According to Smith and Gorski (1985) there are early, middle, and late stages of codependency.[5]

1. "The early stage of codependence is characterized by attempts at normal problem solving that sometimes work but progressively more often fail to work. Alcohol and/or drug use is not specifically identified as the problem and as various problems begin to occur each one is viewed and dealt with as a separate problem. The codependent is invited to believe a sincere delusion: that the alcoholic/addict is a normal user and that the problems are caused by people and things other than the drinking and/or using."

2. "The Middle Stage is characterized by the codependent's loss of personal boundaries. The codependent's boundaries extend to include the alcoholic/addict as a projection of self. The alcoholic's/addict's state of well-being becomes the standard against which she/he measures herself/himself. As a result, the co-dependent develops habitual self-defeating behaviors."

3. "The late stage is characterized by two things: 1) the codependent suffers major physical and emotional problems related to the high stress levels in the family and 2) the codependent makes attempts to withdraw from the alcoholic/addict."

C. Another feature of the codependent is the enabling that supports the behavior or feelings of the codependents. An enabler is anyone who promotes the dependency of another. Characteristics of enabling are:

1. Making excuses.

2. Assuming responsibility for another's actions.

3. Allowing the alcoholic/addict to set *all* family priorities, and everyone's needs in the family are *secondary*.

4. The enabler not only cleans what the codependent messes up but denies it ever happened.

5. The enabler will become financially and emotionally drained by the alcoholic/addict (getting them out of prison or jail).

6. Avoidance is a primary mechanism.

7. Denial is learned by the codependent and is used frequently. The codependent

---

[4]Webster New World Dictionary, pages 378 and 271.

[5]Smith and Gorski, Co-dependent Progression, 1985, The CENAPS Corp., Hazel Crest. IL.

children of codependent adults will learn to rely on denial and lies as the delusion increases and engulfs them.

D. The feelings associated with codependency are:

1. Mistrust and suspicion.

2. Guilt.

3. Fear.

4. Isolation from those who could help.

5. Seem to always be in crisis state.

6. Because of the emotional instability of the relationship, often confused and overwhelmed.

7. Thought patterns become preoccupied with uncertainty of any future activities.

8. Children may be undisciplined, and their education is left to faulty role models experiences and to peer interactions.

E. Nursing interventions

1. Therapeutic communications

a. Be matter of fact.

b. Be a good listener.

c. Redirect patient as needed.

d. Know what is expected of the patient.

e. Do not buy into the delusional system of the patient.

2. Patient activities

a. Identify and examine the codependent relationship.

b. Participate in group activities.

c. Participate in individual psychotherapy.

d. Identify the underlying feelings associated with the codependency.

e. Prepare for the coming separation anxiety of discharge from the milieu.

f. The feelings must emerge to be appropriately dealt with.

S U M M A R Y

Upon completion of Chapter 7 the student will be able to

- Assess the patient for substance abuse.
- Assess patients who are addicted to substances.
- Assist with planning for the interventions related to substance abuse.
- Implement interventions as prescribed by the nursing staff.
- Evaluate the effectiveness of the outcome of interventions.

Review Questions

1. The best definition of an alcoholic is:

   a. A person who regularly consumes alcohol.
   b. A person who regularly goes on "benders", "binges" or "drinking bouts."
   c. A person who drinks to escape from reality.
   d. A person who has developed a psychological dependency to alcohol.

2. The person who is experiencing alcoholic withdrawal is most likely to have which of the following hallucinations:

   a. Visual.
   b. Auditory.
   c. Tactile.
   d. Olfactory.

3. Alcohol is:

   a. A CNS stimulant.
   b. A CNS depressant.
   c. A minor tranquilizer.
   d. A fat oxidizer.

4. The drug that is used specifically to limit alcohol intake is:

   a. Librium.
   b. Chloropromazine.
   c. Antabuse.
   d. Dilantin.

5. You are assessing a patient who was just admitted in acute alcohol detoxification with delirium tremens. Which of the following sets of symptoms would you identify that are related to the delirium tremens?

   a. Manipulation, denial, and negativism.
   b. Confusion, fine muscular tremors, and restlessness.
   c. Depression, withdrawal, and tearfulness.
   d. Suspicion, stubbornness, and unpredictability.

6. The primary site where alcohol is detoxified is:

   a. The intestines.
   b. The liver.
   c. The brain.
   d. The kidneys.

7. The defense mechanisms most commonly used by the alcoholic include all except one of the following:

   a. Sublimation.
   b. Rationalization.
   c. Projection.
   d. Denial.

8. When a patient is taking disulfiram and consumes alcohol in any quantity he/she will likely experience which of the following sets of symptoms?

   a. Elation, grandiosity, and reduced libido.
   b. Nausea, cardiac palpitations, and vomiting.
   c. Severe headaches, dermatitis, and nocturnal sweating.
   d. Gastritis, jaundice, and hallucinations.

9. The most difficult problem in working with those addicted to substances is:

   a. Combating withdrawal symptoms.
   b. Keeping the patient free of all drugs or medications, unless ordered.
   c. Lack of family cooperation.
   d. Teaching the danger of using even stronger drugs.

10. A careful assessment of the drug addict who is expected to have immediate withdrawal symptoms would include which of the following sets of symptoms?

   a. Drowsiness, confusion, mental lability, and hallucinations.
   b. Lacrimation, muscle twitching, rhinorrhea, and insomnia.
   c. Tremors, euphoria, nausea, and cardiac palpitations.
   d. Inappropriate affect, restlessness, and increased libido.

CHAPTER 8

Children and Youth with Emotional Problems

KEY CHAPTER OBJECTIVES

Upon completion of Chapter 8, the student should be able to identify satisfactorily correct answers to questions regarding the following knowledge areas:

- Children and youth who have emotional problems, developmental disorders, and mental health problems.

MENTAL ILLNESS ASSOCIATED WITH CHILDREN AND ADOLESCENTS

The term youth includes the 3-year to 18-year old population.

A. Expected nursing behaviors that will assist with the understanding of emotional needs of children and youth:

1. Communicating.

2. Listening.

3. Empathizing.

4. Recording.

B. Relationship of child and adolescent to the family unit.

1. A strong underpinning of a child is based on a healthy and mutually respectful relationship within the family unit.

a. Rejection, indifference, or total self-reliance may foster rebellious or disturbed behaviors.

b. Children/adolescents observe role models very closely.

c. These patients must be taught limits on behaviors with love and caring so they may comply with standards and rules established by society.

d. If the parents are nurturing and love and support these children and youth, then self-esteem will be enhanced and maintain these children and youth into adulthood.

2. Common family stressors that affect children and youth:

a. Economic factors

1) Both parents work full time.

2) These children will have less contact with their parents.

3) Unlimited independence may be available at an early age. This is before the child is able to manage, in a responsible way, all of the unstructured time.

b. Social factors

1) Evolution of the family structure

a) The high divorce rate (estimated at 50%)

b) A merging of first and second families

c) Single parent homes

c. Psychological factors

1) As parents are adversely affected by life events, they may turn to alcoholism or child abuse, thus directly affecting the child's psyche.

2) The stability of emotional development may be altered by divorce.

3. High-risk children

a. Children faced with traumatic experiences during early years of life, such as death of a parent, may foster the creation of unhealthy coping mechanisms that are used in later life.

  b. The child is immature and impressionable, and operating from a child-based fantasy, and may eventually engage in maladaptive behaviors.

4. Children of divorced parents

  a. From a child's perspective the divorce means:

    1) Break up of family loyalties.

    2) Choosing the parent to live with, or not being given the option to select the parent. The court usually awards custody of the children to whomever it sees fit without regard to the children's choice.

    3) Wishing or dreaming that parents can resolve differences. (Fantasy)

    4) The possibility of the need to reject both parents and live with another family member.

  b. The predivorce period

    1) Living with the stressors that are causing the marital difficulties.

    2) Strong guilt feelings and alienation sometimes emerge.

    3) Listening to the parents argue causes emotional stress, and depending on the nature of the argument may translate into guilt, hate, anger, or rage in the child.

    4) If physical violence occurs, then the child will make a forced choice to either (1) stay out of the way or (2) select the parent to support.

  c. Somatic symptoms may begin to appear, such as:

    1) Nervous twitches.

    2) Change in sleeping patterns.

    3) Change in weight.

    4) Change in nutritional intake.

    5) May be prone to develop ulcers.

    6) May have gastrointestinal changes such as nausea, vomiting, and/or diarrhea.

  d. Psychological changes may be:

    1) Increasing feelings of insecurity.

    2) Regression to a former more comfortable period of development.

    3) Guilt that the child has caused the problem.

    4) May begin acting out or using other attention-seeking behaviors.

  e. Behaviors that may emerge:

    1) Anger

      a) The child will use the defense mechanisms at his/her disposal.

      b) Temper tantrums.

      c) Overobedience.

            d) Blame and shame.

      2) Anxiety

            a) Children worry about the future, etc.

            b) Great fear of abandonment.

            c) Fear of marriage. In later life they may not marry because of the fear that divorce will happen to them.

      3) Guilt

            a) Highest in preschoolers and young school-age children.

            b) Feel that they are personally responsible for the divorce.

      4) Grief

            a) Divorce is viewed by the child as the loss of a parent and possibly, that may be equivalent to the death of a parent.

            b) Grieving behaviors are: depression, withdrawal, and unacceptable patterns of behavior.

      5) Regression

            a) Thumb sucking.

            b) Bed wetting.

            c) Bottle feedings.

            d) Older children may have difficulty with interpersonal relationships and act out based on their feelings of anger, and guilt.

C. Children of parents who are psychiatric patients may have special needs based on the following:

   1. Stressful to the entire family, especially during acute episodes requiring hospitalization.

   2. Separation crisis leading to deprivation of parental care.

      a. There may be disruptions in—

         1) Child care

         2) Health care

         3) Education

      b. Temporary caretakers may cause stress.

      c. Separation anxiety may be evident.

      d. Binding and bonding may be affected.

D. Children of substance abusers

   1. Children will be affected if one or both parents substance abuse.

   2. The role modeling process will be abnormal.

   3. An increased likelihood that the child will be a substance abuser when an adult or will marry a substance abuser.

   4. Children may assume the role of:

    a. The parent.

        1) Learn adult behavior at an early age.

        2) Because of the parenting role, they will be unable to enjoy their own childhood.

        3) Learn to take care of not only themselves, but the rest of the family as well, including the substance abuser.

        4) May delude themselves into believing that their own feelings are not as important as those whom they are trying to nurture.

        5) Learn to deny the substance abusing.

        6) Because substance abuse is the parental role model, children may begin substance abusing to comply/conform to the role model they are being presented.

    b. The family mediator

        1) Must learn to resolve the family disputes.

        2) Learn the signals for the substance abusing and send siblings to a "safe place" while the substance abuse is extremely intense.

        3) May become physically withdrawn and inactive during outbursts of substance abuse.

        4) Eventually believe that they are not in control of their lives.
These may be the beginnings of codependency.

E. Children who are abused.

  1. Abuse and neglect

    a. Physical injury—purposeful acts of bodily injury.

    b. Mental injury—caused by highly personal and threatening, judgmental, or put-down statements. For instance, constantly telling a straight "A" student he/she is dumb or stupid. The parent may also engage in vicious name calling and profanity directed at the child.

    c. Sexual abuse—any sexual contact with a child. *See* pedophilia.

    d. Negligence or neglect.

        1) Emotional negligence may be caused by lack of human interactions.

        2) Physical negligence is associated with depriving the child of physical necessities such as clothes, shoes in the winter; emotional necessities such as love, kindness; nutritional needs such as food, water; and medical needs such as taking the child to a doctor when he/she is ill.

  2. In all states, health care practitioners are *required* to report suspected cases or actual cases of *any* form of abuse.

  3. Because of fear and distrust, it is often very difficult for the child to tell anyone the real truth about the abuse. Gaining a trusting relationship is the first step in identifying the underlying neglect or abuse.

  4. Behaviors associated with abuse are:

        a. Withdrawal.

        b. Passivity.

        c. Lethargy.

        d. Blunted affect.

        e. Regression to an earlier safe time.

        f. Nocturnal enuresis—bed wetting.

        g. Retaining feces, known as encopresis.

        h. Appetite changes such as refusing to eat.

        i. Vomiting

        j. Begins to distrust any touching or physical contact.

        k. Moodiness.

        l. Excessive crying.

        m. Silence.

        n. Poor or no eye contact.

    5. Parents who abuse children

        a. Displace their feelings on children.

        b. Are unable to cope with their own feelings or stressors such as:

           1) Loss of employment

           2) Financial worries

           3) Sudden or abrupt changes in living situation

           4) Substance abuse

        c. Are generally unable to form intimate and sensitive relationships with others.

        d. May have been abused when they were children.

        e. Have inadequate parenting skills.

        f. May be suspicious and distrustful of others.

    6. Types of parents who abuse children are:

        a. Undercontrolled parent who blames child for family problems.

        b. Overcontrolled parent who feels a child's behavior is corrected by punishment.

        c. Parents who are fantasy-prone respond to the fantasy world rather than to the world of reality.

        d. The guilty parent who is disturbed by the abusive treatment of the child may increase the intensity of the abuse.

  F. Nursing interventions of the child at risk.

    1. Learn about children at risk.

    2. Establish a therapeutic relationship with the child and family.

3. Learn to communicate with children at a level that they can understand.

4. Be a child advocate.

5. Identify family members who have undergone or who are undergoing separation, marriage, or divorce. Listen to the child's point of view about the changes in the family.

6. Observe for any family's or individual's stressors such as financial.

7. Review the family's history from the charts.

8. Accurately annotate findings in the patient's medical record(s).

9. Teach the identified family members to use healthy coping skills.

10. Actively support family group activities.

11. Assist in discharge planning.

G. Levels of prevention in supporting high-risk children.

1. Primary prevention

a. The goal is to reduce the occurrences of mental health alterations by helping the family to identify, understand, and manage life stressors.

b. Identify the child or children at risk.

c. The family may need:

1) Child development classes

2) Prenatal classes

3) Prevention of child abuse by social services groups

4) Parenting or child-rearing classes

5) Family therapy

2. Secondary prevention

a. Involves early identification of mental illness to treat the mental disorders.

b. Interventions include, but are not limited to:

1) Team conferences

2) Nursing assessments with planned outcome evaluation

3) Partial or short term hospitalization based on medical decision

3. Tertiary prevention

a. Goals

1) Reduce long-term disability.

2) Assist the patient in returning to a home environment.

b. Interventions

1) Follow-up with outpatient visits.

2) Provide home visits if possible.

3) Participate in family and team discharge planning conferences.

4) Educate the family unit until identified knowledge deficits are corrected.

DEVELOPMENTAL DISORDERS

Mental retardation (MR).

A. General information

1. About 1% of the population is thought to be affected.

2. May be genetic in origin

   a. Down syndrome

   b. Phenylketonuria (PKU)

   c. Galactosemia

   d. Congenital hypothyroidism

3. About 10% of MR results from brain injury or from infection in utero. Approximately 5% of MR is the result of physical disorders such as traumas, infections, and lead poisoning. Approximately 30% results from early alterations in embryonic development. Hereditary factors may account for as much as 5% of MR. Environmental influences, such as social and linguistic deprivation, may account for 15 to 20% of the disorders.[1]

4. The male to female ratio is 1.5:1.

B. Characteristics

1. Less than average intelligence quotient (IQ)

2. Degrees of severity of mental retardation

SEVERITY	IQ
a. Profound	Below 25
b. Severe	20–25 to 35–40
c. Moderate	35–40 to 50–55
d. Mild	50–55 to 70

3. There may be a deficit or at least some degree of impairment in adaptive functioning. Adaptive functioning refers to the person's skills in social skills, communication abilities, and ability to perform activities of daily living.

4. Occurs before the age of 18.

C. Functioning levels/nursing interventions

1. Mild (50–55 to 70)

   a. Are able to develop communication skills during preschool years.

   b. Are usually able to achieve educational skills up to the sixth grade by the time they are in their teens.

   c. As adults, they should be able to support themselves and live independently or with minimal supervision.

   d. Nursing interventions

[1]American Psychiatric Association, DSSM-III-R, 3rd ed., revised, 28–32, 1987.

        1) Support the family.

        2) Assist with the teaching of activities of daily living.

        3) Foster independence.

2. Moderate (35–40 to 50–55)

    a. Are able to develop some communication and social skills.

    b. Unlikely to develop beyond the second grade.

    c. As adults, they will most likely be able to contribute to their own support by performing unskilled or semiskilled work.

    d. These individuals may be able to live independently or may require some degree of supervised living.

    e. Nursing interventions

        1) Support the team approach to the patient's learning of skills.

        2) Assist with and support the independence level achieved.

3. Severe (20–25 to 35–40)

    a. They will most likely learn to talk.

    b. Can be trained usually in only the most rudimentary self-care.

    c. As adults, they will be able to perform simple tasks under supervision.

    d. Nursing interventions

        1) Reinforce previously learned skills.

        2) When performing skills, closely supervise for safety.

4. Profound (below 25)

    a. Have minimal sensorimotor functioning.

    b. Reside in highly structured environment, with direct supervision.

    c. Nursing interventions

        1) Require abundant multiple sensory stimulations.

        2) Be sensitive and therapeutic.[2]

SPECIFIC DEVELOPMENTAL DISORDERS

Autistic Disorder

DEFINITION

AUTISM: A form of thinking. It generally implies that the thoughts and behaviors are derived from the subject her/himself. The behaviors/thoughts may appear in the form of daydreams, fantasies, delusions, hallucinations, etc. This thinking is directed inward to emotions and feelings that result in observed behaviors.[3]

---

[2]Campbell, R., Psychiatric Dictionary, 5th ed., 66, 1981.

[3]Adapted from Campbell, Psychiatric Dictionary, 66.

Autistic features may be based in *behavior, communication, or activities and interests.*

A. Behaviors include any of the following:

    1. The patient has a lack of awareness of the feelings of others.

    2. The patient does not seek comfort at times of distress.

    3. The patient does not imitate.

    4. The patient does not engage in normal social play. Prefers to play without others being present. If someone else is present, they will most likely be ignored.

    5. The patient is unable to make peer relationships.

B. Verbal and nonverbal communication

    1. The autistic person does not communicate at all.

    2. Nonverbal communication is strong when attempts to cause social interactions occur.

    3. The autistic person generally does not engage in activities that require imagination.

    4. When speech is produced, it is abnormal such as high or low pitched or monotone.

    5. The form or content of speech may be repetitive, irrelevant, or both.

    6. The autistic person is unable to initiate or sustain a conversation.

C. Activities and interests

    1. Stereotyped body movements such as spinning or head banging.

    2. The patient has a persistent preoccupation with objects.

    3. The patient may become very distressed if any object in the environment is changed or moved.

    4. Absolutely insists on rigid adherence to the same routine.

    5. The autistic person has a restricted range of interests and a preoccupation with one narrow interest.

Conduct Disorder

A. Characteristics

    1. Persistent patterns of behaviors that violate the basic rights of others.

    2. Occurs at home, in the school, with peers, and in the community.

    3. Physical aggression is common.

    4. Covert (secret) stealing is common.

    5. Physical cruelty to other persons or animals.

    6. Conduct disorder patients may engage in mugging, purse snatching, extortion, or armed robbery.

7. Later, the conduct disorder person may engage in physical violence such as rape, assault, or homicide.

8. Cheating and truancy from school are common.

9. Running away from home is likely.

10. Other behaviors may include:

    a. Using tobacco.

    b. Alcohol.

    c. Substance abuse.

    d. Abnormal sexual behaviors.

    e. Total disregard for the rights and property of others.

    f. No guilt or remorse for violating others.

11. May use weapons to settle disputes.

12. May deliberately set fires.

B. Consequences—outcomes

1. Will be in trouble with law enforcement.

2. As adult will have an antisocial personality disorder.

3. May be able to achieve reasonable social and occupational adjustment.

4. If behavior is out of control and threatens others, then the possibility of hospitalization becomes a reality for this patient.

5. Sexually transmitted diseases (STDs).

6. Unwanted (unplanned) pregnancies.

7. May suffer physical retaliation from others who were violated.

8. Suicide is a possible outcome.

Oppositional Defiant Disorder (ODD)

A. Characteristics

1. Less hostile than Conduct Disorder.

2. Argumentative.

3. Negativism.

4. Defiant behavior toward any authority.

5. The patient blames others for mistakes.

6. Generally obvious at home.

7. Loses temper easily.

8. Cursing, swearing, and profane language are used.

9. Outbursts of anger.

B. The underlying feelings may be:

1. Low self-esteem.

2. Low frustration tolerance.

3. Low self-confidence.

MENTAL HEALTH PROBLEMS OF CHILDREN AND YOUTH

A. The child with depression

1. Emotions

   a. The patient may have a sad affect.

   b. The patient may be experiencing loneliness.

   c. The patient may be experiencing hopelessness due to the inability to set or attain goals.

   d. The patient may be experiencing helplessness because of lack of control.

   e. The patient may convert internal anger into internal rage, which eventually may be externalized anger or rage.

2. Patient behaviors that may precede depression.

   a. Lack of academic achievement.

   b. Lack of social success.

   c. Use of mind-altering substances.

   d. Avoidance of reality.

   e. Anger or rage.

   f. Belligerent or rebellious behavior toward authority: parents, education, or law enforcement.

   g. Running away from problems.

   h. Somatic (physical) symptoms.

      1) Headaches

      2) Stomach aches, nausea, vomiting, or diarrhea

      3) Anorexia

3. Factors that may cause depression.

   a. Divorce.

   b. Death of a relative or significant other.

   c. Acute or chronic illness.

   d. Prolonged separation from significant person(s).

   e. Prepuberty changes.

   f. Changes associated with adolescence.

   g. Lack of peer interaction.

4. Assessing the depressed child or adolescent.

    a. Unexplained or inappropriate crying.

    b. Out of control behavior such as temper tantrums.

    c. Depressed or retarded-appearing motor activities—slow movements.

    d. Pulling one's own hair.

    e. The beginning of self-mutilation behavior; for example, writing name of fantasy boy or girl friend on leg or arm that results in tissue destruction.

    f. Refuses food.

    g. Bed wetting or retaining fecal material.

    h. Neglecting personal appearance with resultant unkempt or disheveled appearance.

    i. Increasing substance abuse.

    j. Suicidal ideation (thoughts) that are verbalized.

5. Nursing interventions

    a. Suicide intervention if self-mutilating or suicidal thinking is in active progress.

    b. Individual psychotherapy.

    c. Group therapy with peers.

    d. Family therapy.

    e. Prescription for medication(s) to resolve the depression.

B. The mentally disturbed child

1. The child who is experiencing internal disorganization of

    a. Perception(s)

    b. Thought(s)

    c. Reality

    d. Judgment

    e. Sense of self

2. Assessment

    a. Not interested in surroundings (environment).

    b. Flat or blunted affect.

    c. Monotone vocalizations.

    d. Quiet, cooperative, submissive, and obedient.

    e. Preoccupied with internal thoughts.

    f. Motion becomes automated.

    g. Seclusive in that the patient chooses to be left alone.

    h. May spend long hours in bed (withdrawn).

    i. May begin to have or to give special meanings to familiar objects or observe ritual behaviors.

    j. May begin to have hallucinations such as:

        1) Auditory

        2) Tactile

        3) Olfactory

        4) Kinesthetic—false sensations of position and posture

    k. Triggered by internal feelings or stimuli.

    l. If hallucinations are present, behaviors you might *objectively* measure include:

        1) Withdrawal and/or seclusion.

        2) Preoccupation—unable to pay attention to the matter at hand.

        3) Inappropriate affect—laughing or crying at an inappropriate time.

        4) Bizarre motor movements—assuming an inappropriate position. Picking an unseen object out of the air.

        5) Interrupted speech.

    m. Delusions

        1) Expresses false beliefs or thoughts and supports them even if proof to the contrary is offered.

        2) The delusions have some basis in reality, but the reality is severely distorted.

        3) Delusions generally do not occur in children under the age of five.

        4) Examples of delusions the patient may have are:

            a) Thoughts are being controlled by an outside force or person.

            b) Thoughts are being transferred (broadcast) to others.

            c) The patient has a total body illness.

            d) May or may not involve religious content.

3. Nursing interventions

    a. Objective observations may include changes in elimination habits, weight loss, bed wetting, or other relevant physical signs.

    b. Assess for behaviors that may indicate the presence of hallucinations.

    c. Plan to assist the patient with personal grooming as needed.

    d. Maintain a therapeutic communication with the patient at all times.

    e. Psychotherapeutic approaches might be:

        1) Individual therapy

        2) Group therapy

        3) Art therapy

        4) Story telling therapy

        5) Relaxation therapy

        6) Family therapy

7) Behavior therapy

8) Biofeedback

9) Sports therapy

10) Reality Oriented Physical Experience Services therapy (ROPES)

11) Milieu therapy

12) Partial or short-term hospitalization

13) Medications to reverse existing symptoms

14) Token economics

DEFINITION

TOKEN ECONOMICS: A technique that is used to assist with control of inappropriate behavior. This consists of earning or giving a certain amount of bargaining ability to the patient for mutually agreed on desired behavior(s). Tokens such as points, marbles, play money may be exchanged for a reward such as a telephone call or a later bed time.

C. The disruptive child.

1. May result from factors such as:

   a. Organic

   b. Social

   c. Cultural

2. Assessing the disruptive child

   a. Disruption of the activities or conversations of others.

   b. Mischievous behavior such as snatching items from others and grinning about it.

   c. Difficulty in taking turns.

   d. Failure in school.

   e. Fidgety.

   f. Frequently threatens others.

   g. Verbal assaults on others.

   h. Destroys others objects without thinking—may become a vandal.

   i. Lies.

   j. Truant from school.

   k. Feels alone and isolated.

3. Nursing interventions

   a. Careful monitoring of diet.

   b. Assist with personal needs such as bathing and hair care.

   c. Assess for wearing of clean clothes.

   d. Monitor for attendance at psychotherapeutic activities as described in "disruptive child."

   e. Use therapeutic communications at all times.

*Note: Because the disruptive child's behavior is so difficult to work with, the parents will
need considerable support and teaching as they are the only source of role modeling
that the child receives.*

D. The adolescent at risk of committing suicide
    1. Can occur in the mentally healthy as well as the mentally ill adolescent.
    2. Once a suicide has been accomplished in a high school group, it is likely that others may also commit suicide, either as a cluster or the result of a suicide pact.
    3. Indicators of impending adolescent suicide:
        a. Extreme despair.
        b. Prolonged depression.
        c. Change in sleeping patterns.
        d. Change in eating patterns.
        e. Undefined problems with grades in school.
        f. Heavy use of drugs.
        g. Unusual behavior such as reckless driving.
        h. Vacant stare.
        i. Begins to verbalize suicidal thoughts.

Always presume verbalization about suicide as a pending suicide and immediately begin an intervention!

        j. Patients tend to be tearful—very sad.
        k. Preoccupied with sad thoughts.
        l. May give significant items to friends—an attempt to settle their "estate."

MILIEU THERAPY

A. Children (ages 3 or 4 to 11 or 12).
    1. Structure of the milieu
        a. Highly structured.
        b. Closely supervised.
        c. Extreme behavior disturbances such as disruptive behaviors.
        d. May require frequent seclusion or personal restraining.
    2. Children are expected to participate in:
        a. Family therapy
        b. Education at the appropriate level

       c. Process group therapy

       d. Social skills therapy

       e. Cooking group

       f. Expressive/receptive language

       g. Recreational therapy

   3. Goals associated with the children's program

       a. Develop a positive self-image.

       b. Develop appropriate social skills.

       c. Improve or increase learning potential.

       d. Develop citizenship qualities.

       e. Prepare for entry into the world of work.

       f. Develop and practice sound personal hygiene.

       g. Develop a creative and effective use of time.

B. Adolescence (ages 10 or 11 to 18).

   1. Substance abuse

       a. Polysubstance abuse (many different substances used simultaneously) is probably the most common admitting diagnosis for the adolescent substance abuser.

       b. Since these patients are admitted by parents, guardians, or the court, their rights are viewed differently, but they still have full force and effect as an adult would.

       c. The patients and the milieu should be free of any mind-altering substances.

       d. The detoxification for the adolescent is as intense as it is for the adult.

   2. Activities that adolescents may be a part of are:

       a. Meditation and goal-setting group

       b. Sober living group

       c. Attends daily step education group; such as 12-step support groups (AA, NA)

       d. Focus or lecture group

       e. Music group

       f. Psychodrama

       g. Reflections group

       h. Individual psychotherapy

       i. Attends school—when in session

       j. Reality Oriented Physical Experience Services (ROPES)

       k. Recreational and occupational therapy

       l. Stress management

       m. All activities of daily living

   3. Patient responsibilities.

a. Maintain appropriate behavior.

b. Be honest and direct.

c. Adhere to the rules of token economics. There will most likely be a system of rewards for good behavior and consequences for inappropriate behaviors. Generally these are based on a system of chips, tokens, or other objects that are given significance by staff and patients.

d. Tell those caring for her/him about any health problems that are experienced.

e. Respect the rights of other patients and staff.

f. Observe the confidentiality of other patients.

g. Keep appointments and cooperate with staff to assure continuity of care.

h. Complete all reading and writing assignments on time.

i. Observe the schedule of events as related to waking and sleeping hours.

4. General guidelines for the adolescent unit.

a. No use of any mind altering drugs or substances

b. No smoking

c. No fighting

d. No fraternization by gender (pairing off)

e. No property damage

f. No profanity or cursing

g. Patients are expected to get to activities on time

h. Patients are expected to participate in all unit activities

i. Patients are not allowed to be in another patient's room

j. No loitering at the nurses desk

k. No food and/or drink are allowed in the patient's room

l. Patients are expected to clean their own rooms and make their own beds

m. Patients may not share clothing or make-up

n. Patients may not give another patient a haircut

o. Visit with their family at the appointed time(s)

5. Objectives of the adolescent psychiatric program are:

a. Provide patient and family with an orientation to the program.

b. Develop new coping skills.

c. Develop a community (milieu) of individuals who work together to help themselves and others.

d. Develop a supportive and caring environment.

e. Develop new listening and communication skills.

f. Develop constructive feedback and reflective techniques.

g. Develop creative problem-solving skills.

h. Develop self-enhancing behaviors.

6. Activities that the adolescent psychiatric patient may participate in are:

a. School

b. Individual therapy

c. Group psychotherapy

d. Cognitive group

e. Psychodrama

f. Trauma group

g. Problem-solving groups

h. Pass goals group

i. Creative arts and crafts

j. Daily goals group

k. Goal reflection group

l. Family therapy

m. Multifamily group

n. Program counseling

o. Therapeutic pass

p. Family weekend

The milieu structure is similar to that of the adolescent with substance abuse.

S U M M A R Y

At the completion of Chapter 8, the student should be able to prepare a plan of care that contains the following essential components in accordance with the APIE format. The APIE format refers to the following competencies:

- Contributes to the assessment component of the care plan by collecting subjective and objective data.
- Assists with preparation of a plan of care.
- Assists with the implementation of nursing care.
- With assistance from the professional nurse, is able to evaluate care and outcome of the plan of care related to patients in each of the following:

> Children and youth (adolescent)at high risk for emotional problems, developmental disorders, and mental retardation

> Specific Development Disorders

> Autistic disorders

> Disorders limiting scholastic development

> Mental health problems of children and youth.

Review Questions

1. The primary goal during the intervention of a child/adolescent patient who is in crisis is:

   a. Stop the abuse.
   b. Let the patient talk.
   c. Try to identify the underlying cause of the crisis.
   d. Stop the crisis.

2. Using token economics, related to behavior is:

   a. Legal.
   b. Bribery.
   c. A form of reward for appropriate behavior.
   d. A form of control given to parents.

3. The best definition of anorexia nervosa is:

   a. A loss of weight.
   b. An increase in appetite.
   c. A decrease in appetite.
   d. A unrealistic overconcern about weight.

4. Which of the following best describes bulimia:

   a. Bingeing, purging to lose weight.
   b. Bingeing only.
   c. Most frequently seen in boys.
   d. Equally common in boys and girls.

5. A suicide pact is:

   a. A way to get even with authority.
   b. Peer decision-based mutual agreement.
   c. A written contract spelling out the terms and conditions of suicide.
   d. Always occurs in disgruntled groups.

6. Which of the following is the correct IQ numbers associated with moderate mental retardation?

   a. 10–15.
   b. 30–35.
   c. 35–55.
   d. 60–70.

7. The best definition of autism is:

   a. Inward directed thinking.
   b. Outward directed thinking.
   c. No behavior of any kind.
   d. On-going wild flurries of behavior.

8. Feelings of depression may lead to feelings of hopelessness. Feelings of hopelessness may lead to feelings of:

   a. Elation.
   b. Rage.

      c. Anorexia.

      d. Suicide.

9. The primary cause of rebellion or disturbed behavior in youth (children and adolescents) is:

      a. Giving an allowance with expected responsibility.

      b. Limiting play hours with others of the same age (peer group).

      c. Limiting amount of television to no more than 1 hour per day.

      d. Parental rejection and/or indifference.

10. No one is certain how much youth neglect/abuse occurs. It is law that:

      a. Physicians must report any abuse.

      b. Nurses must report any abuse.

      c. Anyone who suspects youth abuse is required to report it.

      d. Only health care workers must report youth abuse.

The Aging Process and Mental Illness

KEY CHAPTER OBJECTIVES

Upon completion of Chapter 9, the student should be able to identify satisfactorily correct answers to questions regarding the following knowledge areas:

- Organic mental disorders
- Polysubstance abuse
- The aging process and mental health

ORGANIC MENTAL DISORDERS [CHARACTERISTICS FROM DSM-III-R]

A. The mentally healthy elderly

1. Characteristics

   a. They have a zest for living.

   b. Productive.

   c. Engaged in social, educational, and cultural events.

   d. Participate in community activities.

   e. Recognize and resolve that whatever they have done with their lives, must now be accepted.

   f. Competent.

   g. Generally independent.

   h. Form a significant segment of societal population.

   i. Ability to cope with problems of daily living.

2. Problems of the elderly

   a. Acute and chronic illness.

   b. Transportation less and less accessible.

   c. Nutrition.

   d. Medication.

   e. Shopping.

   f. Abuse.

   g. Decreasing sensory functions.

   h. Income is usually fixed.

3. Resources available

   a. Community nursing service.

   b. Home aids and home health

   c. Limited transportation to:

      1) Shopping

      2) Businesses

      3) Physicians

      4) Church

      5) Social events

   d. Meals on Wheels

   e. Dietary education and menu planning assistance.

   f. Monitoring of medications by community health nurse.

   g. Surveys of living quarters for presence or absence of safety hazards.

B. Organic mental disorders[1]

  1. Early signs

    a. Losing things

    b. Making money errors

    c. Inefficiency at work

    d. Mixing up or missing appointments

    e. Decrease in social skills

    f. Easily tires

    g. Forgetful

  2. Later signs

    a. Appearance becomes disheveled by neglect.

    b. May become incontinent of bladder and/or bowels.

    c. Unable to accept new ideas.

    d. Disorientation to new settings.

    e. Apathetic.

  3. Organic delusional syndrome

    a. May experience delusions.

    b. May be related to use of amphetamines, alcohol, and/or cocaine.

    c. Organic affective syndrome

      1) Mood disturbance.

      2) Related to amphetamines and hallucinogens.

      3) Organic disorders associated with circulatory disturbances.

      4) Cerebro-vascular accident (CVA) — ischemia or infarcts.

      5) Transient ischemic attacks (TIA).

      6) Senile dementia.

        a) Chronic, typically irreversible impairment of intellectual functioning.

        b) If this occurs before 65, it may be diagnosed as Alzheimer's.

        c) Huntington's chorea.

      7) Focal cerebral disorders.

        a) Symptoms are dependent on the area of the cerebrum that is involved.

        b) May be localized or generalized.

      8) Organic mental disorders induced by drugs or poisons.

        a) Causes changes in perception, attention and thought processes.

        b) Sedatives and hypnotics are associated with 50% of these disorders.

---

[1]DSM-III-R, 3rd ed., Rev., 97–163, 1987

C. Delirium

1. Inability to maintain attention to external stimuli

2. Disorganized thinking

   a. Rambling speech

   b. Irrelevant or incoherent speech

3. Reduced level of consciousness

4. Sensory misperceptions

5. Disturbed sleeping patterns

6. Disorientation to time, place, or person

7. Memory impairment

8. Usually rapid onset

D. Dementia

1. Intellectual defects

2. Interference with social and occupational functioning

3. Impaired memory

4. May become impulsive

5. May begin to show lack of emotional control

6. Will lack the ability to solve problems

7. Unable to think in the abstract

8. Personality changes may occur

9. Severity of dementia is measured as mild, moderate, or severe

E. Amnestic syndrome

1. Impairment of short- and long-term memory.

2. May be disorientated to time, place, or person.

3. Confabulation may be present. (Confabulation is the filling in of details with imagined events.)

4. Affect may become flat.

5. Apathy may be present.

F. Organic hallucinosis

1. Persistent or recurring hallucinations. The hallucinations may be auditory, visual, sensory, or gustatory depending on the specific organic factor.

2. The hallucinations may be very powerful and lead to depression.

3. The patient may have tremendous anxiety related to the hallucinations.

G. Organic delusional syndrome

1. Syndrome is delusion-based

2. Tends to occur in a normal state of consciousness due to a specific organic factor

3. Mild cognitive (perception of the world around us) impairment

    4. May be disoriented to place, time, person, and purpose

    5. Speech may be incoherent (doesn't make sense)

    6. Mood may be dysphoric (a generalized, vague feeling of illness)

    7. May not be able to function socially

    8. May not be able to function in patient's occupation

    9. Motor activity is labile—either increased or decreased

H. Organic mood syndrome

    1. Disturbance in mood

    2. May be manic

    3. May be in a depressive mood

    4. May be mixed, or in both manic and depressive mood cycle

    5. Cause is a specific organic factor

I. Organic anxiety syndrome

    1. Recurrent panic attacks

    2. May have generalized anxiety

    3. Occurs in a normal conscious state

    4. May be related to endocrine disorder

    5. May be related to substance intoxication or withdrawal from substances

    6. Brain tumors may be the underlying pathologic cause.

J. Organic personality syndrome

    1. Labile affect—varying from depression to euphoria

    2. Overt aggression

    3. Rage reactions

    4. Impaired social judgment

    5. Apathy

    6. Suspicion and paranoid ideation

    7. Impaired social judgment

    8. Explosive outbursts

    9. Sexual indiscretions

K. Substance abuse

    1. All symptoms are related to recent ingestion of a psychoactive substance.

    2. The symptoms are substance-specific; that is, each substance ingested carries with it its own set of symptoms.

    3. The substances offer a variety of side effects such as altering mind functioning, thought processes, seeking attention, withdrawal, and emotional controls.

L. Withdrawal from substance abuse

    1. Withdrawal begins when the ingestion of the substance stops.

    2. Common withdrawal symptoms:

a. Anxiety.

b. Restlessness.

c. Irritable.

d. Gastrointestinal symptoms (nausea, vomiting, and anorexia).

e. Insomnia.

f. Inability to focus on the task at hand.

M. Substances most frequently abused

1. Alcohol

2. Amphetamines

3. Caffeine

4. Cannabis

5. Cocaine

6. Hallucinogens

7. Inhalants—paints, etc.

8. Nicotine

9. Opiates

10. Phencyclidine (PCP)

11. Sedatives

12. Hypnotics

13. Anxiolytics

14. Benzodiazapines, i.e., Valium

N. Alzheimer's disease

1. Cause is not known, but may be a combination of genetic predisposition. Down's syndrome predisposes to Alzheimer's disease

2. Advancing age

3. Behaviors associated with Alzheimer's disease

a. Depends on the areas of the brain that are involved. This is a highly selective process within the structure of the brain.

b. Cognitive (perceptive abilities) may be affected.

c. Memory may be disturbed.

d. Inability to think abstractly.

e. Lack of impulse control.

f. Judgment becomes less appropriate.

g. Personality may be disturbed.

h. Delirium, delusions, and/or depression may be present.

O. Multi infarct dementia.

1. Causes may be one or more of the following:

       a. Vascular disease

       b. Arterial hypertension

       c. Cerebral hypoxia

       d. Hypoglycemia

       e. Cerebral embolism

    2. Behaviors associated with multi infarct dementia

       a. Onset is abrupt

       b. Disturbances in memory

       c. Disturbances in abstract thinking

       d. Alterations in impulse control

       e. Personality may change

       f. There may also be neurological deficits of extremities.[2]

P. Treatment is directed at:

    1. Elimination of the physical cause, if known.

    2. Removal of drugs, if drug-induced.

    3 Many may not have an effective treatment.

Q. Places of treatment of the mentally ill

    1 Nursing homes.

    2. Geriatric centers.

    3. Psychiatric facilities.

    4. Foster care in private homes.

    5. Day care centers

    6. Clubs or other community resources.

R. Nursing interventions

    1. Maintain dignity of the individual.

    2. Promote independence.

    3. Offer friendship.

    4. Assure patient safety by adjusting milieu for visual and hearing deficits.

    5. Be alert to potential suicide.

    6. Observe nutritional intake.

    7. Provide opportunities for social interactions (for instance, grooming) to occur outside the unit.

    8. Reality therapy as needed.

    9. Assess elimination—both urine and bowel.

---

[2]DSM-III-R, 3rd ed., Rev., 121, 1987

10. Take time with these patients.

11. Maintain a safe milieu (environment).

S. Activities for the institutionalized patient

1. Reminiscence sessions

2. Religious activities

3. Exercise groups

4. Social activities

5. Leisure activities

6. Therapeutic activities

7. Rehabilitation services

SUMMARY

Upon completing Chapter 9, the student will be able to:
promote therapeutic communications in the geriatric–psychiatric milieu.

1. Be able to assess for physical–mental illness.
2. Assist with planning interventions for the aging patient.
3. Safely provide interventions for the aging patient.
4. Assist with evaluating the outcome of care given.

Review Questions

1. Mental processes and behaviors that serve to protect our self-esteem by reducing the anxieties encountered in everyday life are called:
   a. General adaptation.
   b. Psychological adaptation.
   c. Defense mechanisms.
   d. Stress reactors.

2. A senile patient is withdrawn and very negative. Which of the following would be the most therapeutic approach to initiating an interaction with the patient?
   a. "Would you like to go to your room where you can be alone?"
   b. "I need a partner to play checkers with me."
   c. "Your family will be terribly disappointed if you do not go to occupational therapy."
   d. "Your doctor wants you to participate in all the activities you can tolerate."

3. Which of the following statements is most true about the aging process?
   a. People age at the same rate.
   b. Aging begins at 65.
   c. Aging begins at 75.
   d. Aging varies at an individual rate.

4. One of the basic attitudes about aging that is prevalent in our hemisphere is that:
   a. The elderly should be held in high esteem.
   b. Since they have already made their contribution to society, their importance has diminished.
   c. Their opinions should be sought out.
   d. They have valuable skills.

5. If an elderly patient complains that "everyone is sure mumbling these days," which of the following is most likely correct?
   a. He/she is just being cranky.
   b. He/she is probably becoming emotionally disturbed.
   c. Her/his hearing may be less acute.
   d. He/she needs a hearing aid.

6. Nurses must come to an understanding of their own feelings about the aging so that:
   a. They can project their feelings to others.
   b. They can be more therapeutic.
   c. They can more easily identify with the ills of the elderly.
   d. They are more interested in their patients.

7. The elderly person will probably eat better if:
   a. Food servings are large.
   b. Offered only high fiber foods.
   c. The foods are liquified or pureed.
   d. Food servings are smaller.

8. A prime consideration for safety when caring for the elderly patient is:
   a. Confine the patient to a small area.
   b. Keep their clothing loose fitting and long.
   c. Provide adequate lighting.
   d. Use open heaters in the bathroom for extra warmth.

9. The most common accidents that involve the elderly are:
   a. Falls.
   b. Burns.
   c. Cuts.
   d. Head trauma.

10. The primary cause of Alzheimer's disease is thought to be:
    a. Schizophrenia.
    b. Substance abuse.
    c. Genetic.
    d. Unknown.

Therapeutic Plans and Treatment

KEY CHAPTER OBJECTIVES.

Upon completion of Chapter 10, the student should be able to identify satisfactorily correct answers to questions regarding the following knowledge areas:

- Treatment plans
- Milieu therapy
- Special milieu

THE TREATMENT PLAN

During the admission, a preliminary treatment plan is written by the professional nurse. This plan may be called preliminary or interim, but it is a temporary plan until the rest of the treatment team has had an opportunity to formulate a comprehensive treatment plan that includes all of the modalities available to the patient. The comprehensive treatment plan may also be named the master treatment plan.

The primary components of the treatment plan are:

- A substantiated medical diagnosis
- A listing of patient strengths or assets
- Long-range goals
- Short-term goals
- Responsibilities of each team member
- Responsibilities listed by modality

All modalities that are a part of the patient's treatment should appear in the treatment plan along with the patient problem(s) that they intend to address.

The goals should be objective, measurable, and contain a target time frame for completion.

Adjunctive Therapy (Modalities)

These are modalities used in the treatment of the mentally ill. There are a number of treatments available to the mental health patient. Before any treatment is instituted, there must be a written physician order. Basically, the treatments can be divided into two groups of patient-centered activities. The first group of activities is specific for the described (medically diagnosed) disorder. The second and equally important group of activities is associated with the milieu.

In this chapter we discuss briefly these two groups of treatments.

Examples of treatments are:

- Electroconvulsive (ECT) therapy, also known as electroseizure therapy and electroshock (EST) therapy.
- Insulin shock therapy
- Family therapy
- Group therapy
- Hydrotherapy
- Behavior modification
- Remotivation therapy
- Reality therapy
- Recreational therapy
- ROPES (reality-oriented physical experience services)

- Occupational therapy
- Psychoactive medications
- Psychoanalysis
- Psychodrama
- Psychotherapy

Electroconvulsive Therapy, Electroseizure Therapy, or Electroshock Therapy

A. Theories of why ECT (EST) works.

1. Permits the patients to forget about painful life experiences.
2. Patients perceive ECT (EST) as a form of punishment and thus improve after treatment because they feel they have been punished for their actions, "I've paid for my sins, and I feel much better."
3. Disrupts the behaviors associated with depressive disorder.
4. Procedure may have the effect of death→rebirth→forgiveness.
5. Allows for primitive movements such as fetal positioning and grunting.

B. Tests completed before ECT (EST).

1. A complete physical examination.
2. Thorough psychological examination.
3. An electrocardiogram (EKG).
4. Chest (posterior/anterior and lateral) and spinal x-rays.
5. Electroencephalogram (EEG).
6. Any other tests or examinations the physician deems appropriate.

C. Patients most likely to benefit from ECT (EST):

1. Depressed patients.
2. Those suffering from prolonged melancholia.

D. Before to the procedure

1. Consent form is signed if the patient is a voluntary admission.
2. Court must agree to ECT (EST) if patient is an involuntary admission.
3. NPO.
4. Be sure that the patient empties bladder just before the procedure.
5. Preanesthesia medications may need to be given if ordered.
6. Remove all metal objects from the patient. The electric current could cause heating of metal objects that could burn the patient. Another possibility is that the items could be misplaced during or after the procedure.
7. Remove any removable objects in the mouth such as partial, dentures; these should be documented if not removed. Check the local policy and procedure manual.

    8. Contact lenses are either removed or left in place at the discretion of the anesthetist.

E. The ECT (EST) treatment

    1. All equipment should be present and checked to make certain that it is functioning properly.

       a. An EST machine.

       b. Oxygen equipment.

       c. Emergency cart.

    2. Nursing staff experienced in ECT (EST) should be present.

    3. The patient should lie on a suitable table or stretcher that is stable enough to support a grand mal seizure, and with adequate properly applied safety devices in place.

    4. The temporal lobe area of the head should be cleaned with appropriate solution(s).

    5. Special electrode paste is applied to the cleaned areas before the electrodes are applied.

    6. Cardiac monitoring devices are placed.

    7. After the medications are given, an airway is established.

    8. The patient will experience a grand mal seizure, varying from mild to severe depending on the amount and effects of the musculoskeletal medications given in combination with the selected anesthetic agents.

    9. There is a recovery period from the anesthesia and muscle relaxants that are given during the procedure which requires that the patient be closely monitored.

    10. A trained staff should stay with the patient until he/she is fully conscious and vital signs are stable.

F. Posttreatment

    1. Liquids are usually given, with progress to diet as tolerated after the gag reflex returns.

    2. Resumes usual diet as tolerated.

    3. Patient may require "line of sight" observations during the confused or disoriented phases of recovery.

    4. A mild analgesic may be given for the post-ECT (EST) headache(s) if so prescribed.

    5. Nurse should offer reassurances and support the patient.

    6. Reality orientation may be necessary.

    7. There will be a period of amnesia.

G. General information to the patient could include:

    1. No pain, muscles may be sore, stiff and there may or may not be an accompanying headache.

    2. The procedure is safe in that there will only be enough electricity to cause a seizure, not enough to kill.

3. It is not possible is to be electrocuted.

4. The number of treatments may vary depending on the state of depression. Usually eight to twelve treatments may be needed. The physician will advise the patient on this point.

5. The confusion that occurs will go away.

6. In several weeks, as memory returns, most of the self-depreciation, sadness, and guilt feelings will probably have dissipated.

H. Provide support by listening to the patient's expression of fear concerning the procedure.

I. Assure patient that he/she will not be alone during the treatment.

J. Reorient the patient after the procedure, and reassure that the feelings of confusion will subside.

K. Observe and record the patient's responses to the treatment.

Insulin Shock (Coma) Therapy

A. Used infrequently in the treatment of schizophrenia.

B. Carefully observe patient for signs and symptoms of insulin shock after treatment.

Family Therapy

A. Type of group therapy involving the patient and her/his family members coming together for the resolution of mutually shared problems.

B. Purposes

1. Assist family members to identify one another's needs.

2. To provide an opportunity to resolve family conflicts or shared anxieties.

3. To develop or reestablish appropriate role relationships.

4. Assist family members in coping with conflict that is occurring within the family unit.

5. To promote a healthy emotional environment allowing for family growth.

6. To enable the family to solve its own problems.

Group Therapy

A. Involves the meeting and directing of several patients, usually in a closed setting. Group is conducted by a therapist or co-therapists.

B. Purposes:

1. Provide a setting in which the respective members of the group may gain insight into thoughts, feelings, and behaviors.

2. Allow the members of the group to provide support during the individual investigations of inner feelings and emotions.

   a. Provide peer input into needed behavioral changes (different perspectives).

   b. Form new and meaningful relationships.

   c. Provide a therapeutic milieu in which patients can freely and openly discuss the demands reality (society) places on them.

   d. Group discussions, using dynamic approaches, aides the patient in achieving goals.

C. Types of groups

   1. Problem-solving groups. From a list of problems generated by the members, the group sets about solving these problems either individually or in smaller independent groups.

   2. Remotivation groups. A planned group situation of patients and nursing staff in which the patients are encouraged to discuss topics that are most meaningful to them. In these groups, the positive aspects of experiences are explored. To instill a sense of future good experiences for the patient to look forward to.

   3. Reality therapy. Assists the patient in rejecting irresponsible behavior and learning new and more socially acceptable behaviors. Reality therapy focuses on current behavior patterns.

   4. Personality reconstruction groups. Taking the personality components and reconstructing them with, for example, new defense mechanisms for better coping and therefore, better adapting to the environment.

   5. Behavior modification. The systematic application of learning principles to change undesired, disruptive, and maladaptive patterns of behavior. When the behavior is improved or is more appropriate, it is rewarded.

   6. A variety of support groups.

D. Hydrotherapy. Using warm, tepid, or cold water or packs, either intermittently or continuously to stimulate or sedate the patient.

E. Recreation therapy. The purpose of recreation therapy is to restructure the patient's daily life around something constructive and offer a balance to the many sedentary groups of the day. Recreation therapy is designed to foster a sense of creative play appropriate to the level of function of the patient. The goal is to provide activities that are fun and afford opportunities for learning. Participation in games or sports by patients and nursing staff to provide physical activity for release of physical pent-up energy, and personal contact in a closer to normal setting. Recreation therapy occurs in a variety of settings, such as picnics, swimming pool activity, gymnasium events, bowling, and other organized unit activities.

F. Reality-oriented physical experience services (ROPES). A form of physical challenge group therapy consisting of a tall vertical challenge surface wherein each patient must learn to trust and rely on a peer for a successful climb. The primary goal is to place individuals in physically, emotionally, and intellectually demanding situations where skills of cooperative problem solving, goal setting, and self-awareness are rapidly developed. Each ROPES event encourages participants to deal with an issue in the here and now, i.e., problems communicating with another or a need to feel successful. The climb may be followed by a slide for life. The typical ROPES course has both high and low elements.

G. Occupational therapy. Active patient participation in useful, constructive, and/or artistic activities within the hospital setting; sometimes referred to as art therapy.

H. Psychoactive medications (*see* Chapter 11).

I. Psychoanalysis. An in-depth analysis of feelings that is conducted by a psychiatrist.

J. Psychodrama. A technique wherein patients are assigned roles to act out. These roles are related to an underlying patient problem.

K. Psychotherapy. Usually individual, where the patient discusses, describes any situation that he/she chooses to talk about. Psychotherapy may be conducted by a psychologist, psychiatrist. or other appropriately credentialed staff.

L. Chemical dependency groups. The groups discuss topics on a variety of subjects in dealing with the dependency disorder(s). The goal being that of increased awareness and education of chemical-dependent patients.

THE MILIEU

A. Milieu therapy—the therapeutic community is defined as "a scientific manipulation of the environment aimed at producing changes in the personality and behavior of the patient."[1]

B. Milieu is a French word meaning total environment.

1. Physical surroundings

2. Staff members

3. Specific programs

C. Purposes:

1. Assist the patient to function within the least restrictive area.

2. Provide a structure for appropriate functioning.

3. Encourage the patient to improve behavior.

4. Assist the patient to regain self-confidence.

5. Enable the patient to reclaim and/or resume responsibility for self.

6. Allow for structure within which socializing skills are effectively increased.

7. Offer the patient protection from self-injury.

D. Characteristics of the milieu.

1. The milieu is a highly interactive environment.

2. The milieu has a group of professionals known as the multidisciplinary team.

3. Provides therapy in a structured setting.

4. Is safe and secure.

---

[1]Psychiatric Dictionary, Campbell, 5th ed., Oxford University Press, New York, 649, 1981.

5. Provides support to patients during periods or episodes of crisis, especially those emotional crises that evolve into physical compromise.

6. Promotes identification of previous unhealthy experiences.

7. Provides an outlet for what would be socially unacceptable behaviors.

8. Expand or contract therapy to an appropriate therapeutic level for the patient.

9. Arrive at mutually agreed upon goals for reentry into the community setting.

10. Personal conduct should always be acceptable.

Specific Milieus

A. Types of patient units

  1. Open

    a. Not locked; used in the case of partial care or convalescing patients.

    b. Patients receive medications, assistance with care, and some therapy depending on need.

    c. Patients work away from the facility but receive counseling before and after work.

    d. For partial care patients, therapy may be given during the day and they return home at night.

  2. Closed

    a. Locked for the safety and protection of the acutely ill patient.

    b. Requires more staff; these patients are at high risk, and therefore, require continuous monitoring and observations.

  3. Partial (hospitalization) care. Therapy occurs primarily during daytime hours or may be extended into the evening hours. Patients return to their own living quarters for the night.

B. Adult milieu

  1. Substance abuse

    a. Provide a safe environment in which the patient may safely detoxify.

    b. Adequate monitoring to prevent physiologic collapse.

    c. Provide medication, if ordered by the physician, to curtail the most harmful physical effects of detoxification.

    d. Correct the underlying nutritional deficits.

    e. Maintain sobriety.

    f. Intervene in the drug-seeking habits of the patient.

    g. Provide an environment to foster treating the underlying cause of the addiction.

    h. Assist the patient to invest in the development of an adequate support group.

2. What the substance abuse patient can expect.

   a. Intense individual psychotherapy to identify the underlying causes of the addiction.

   b. Rigorous adherence to the structure within the program of learning about substance abuse and addiction.

   c. Responsibility for self.

   d. Learning to make decisions that are compatible with a healthy lifestyle. See psychiatric adult patient expectations.

C. Psychiatric milieu. A milieu that is specifically designed and staffed to care for those patients with primarily psychiatric disorders.

1. Young adults (ages 18 to 30).

   a. Mental illness in this group is generally attributed to a failed or flawed maturation process.

   b. Unresolved problems or residual problems from earlier years seem to become accentuated.

   c. The emergence of psychiatric disorders such as schizophrenia, unipolar and bipolar affective disorders, and severe personality disorders.

   d. Many of these young patients can be treated successfully in inpatient settings; however, others will require periodic reassessment and subsequent hospitalization.

2. Midlife adults (ages 30 to 50).

   a. Psychiatric disorders may be primarily from anxiety and depressive life events.

   b. Life-threatening despair; depression may lead to thoughts of self-destruction.

   c. Patients seem to benefit from hospitalization initially, and then follow-up in a partial care setting.

   d. During hospitalization, the concentrated focus of treatment is on the multidisciplinary team combined with psychotherapeutic medications, and the safety and security of the patient in the milieu. This combination yields a tremendously effective treatment.

3. Older adults (ages 50 to 65).

   a. The earlier anxieties and despairs in the older patient combined with the aging process may produce profound depressive episodes.

   b. The incidence of suicide, both the planning and the execution of the act, are more likely to occur.

4. Admission to the psychiatric unit

   a. The patient poses a clear, active threat to self or others.

   b. The patient is impaired (mental disorder) to such a degree that he/she is unable to interact in social, familial, and/or occupational settings

    c. The patient requires continuous skilled observation only available in a hospital.

    d. The patient lacks the support of an appropriate external social system.

    e. The patient requires intensive treatment for both emotional and/or behavioral components of psychiatric disorders.

5. What the adult psychiatric patient may expect

    a. Treatment that will be determined by the treatment team.

    b. A safe milieu.

    c. Unit rules that provide a clear structure.

    d. A level or phase system that affords opportunity to advance in responsibilities as soon as practicable.

    e. A sense of community.

    f. A shared, mutual respect for each individual.

    g. Beneficial interactions and development of relationships with other patients and staff.

6. General characteristics of the adult psychiatric unit

    a. All time spent is in the interest of achieving specific therapeutic goals.

    b. Patients are expected to take responsibility for their own behaviors and regain power over their own lives.

    c. Affords opportunity to solve problems with positive feedback.

    d. Learning from mistakes is important, therefore, risk-taking is important.

    e. Learn to verbalize feelings appropriately and accept feedback regarding behaviors.

    f. Learn to function autonomously.

    g. Learn about human relationships and engage in these relationships.

    h. Patients to be directed or redirected into reality.

    i. Instill a sense of order and justice.

    j. Afford the patient protection from danger to self, others, or the environment.

7. Methods used by staff to deal with inappropriate behaviors include, but are not limited to:

    a. Extinction—withholding attention for negative behavior.

    b. Providing direction—providing alternatives that are more likely to be successful in meeting patient needs.

    c. Setting limits—generally used when direction does not result in a (fairly immediate) behavior change. A clear and concise statement is made to the patient as to what behavior is not appropriate along with the suggestions of which behaviors are most appropriate.

    d. Verbal reprimands—a two-part statement that informs the patient of the inappropriate behavior, but includes consequences if the inappropriate behavior continues.

    e. Privilege removal—modifies inappropriate behavior by removing a privilege that is specifically associated with the inappropriate behavior.

    f. Time out—patient or staff initiate disruption of behaviors. This allows the patient time to consider the behavior by removing him/herself from a stimulating environment.

> **CAUTION**: NEVER ATTEMPT TO IMPOSE ANY OF THESE TECHNIQUES UNLESS THE REST OF STAFF IS AWARE! THIS IS TERMED THE UNITED FRONT APPROACH.

8. What the psychogeriatric patient may expect while hospitalized.

    a. Nursing care appropriate to the level of need; assistance with activities of daily living.

    b. Medications as prescribed by the physician.

    c. Treatment that may include, but is not limited to, therapies such as group, topic group, family, activities, and psychotherapy.

    d. Expected to participate in community meetings, positive strokes, phase system and advancement in phase system, patient government, and other scheduled activities.

9. Patient responsibilities during hospitalization.

    a. Participate in all scheduled patient activities according to the published schedules.

    b. Maintain the cleanliness of personal clothing.

    c. Laundry may be used at times other than scheduled therapeutic activities.

    d. Observe the clean linen schedule.

    e. At the appropriate times, the patients are expected to attend meals at the appointed place.

    f. Availability of healthy snacks.

    g. If the patient is ordered on a special diet, he/she should make this known in the dining room to the staff serving the meal.

    h. Observe the rules of the use of the telephone.

    i. Observe wake up and bedtime rules.

    j. Make themselves knowledgeable about visiting hours, mailing letters, and storage of valuables.

    k. Use the Day Room area as appropriate.

    l. Be aware of the criteria for therapeutic assignments (passes).

D. Suggested topics for orientation of the nurse entering the mental health setting.

    1. Introduction to the facility.

    2. Confidentiality.

    3. Patients' rights.

4. Patient abuse and neglect.

5. Emergency and safety procedures.

6. Employment description or student evaluation.

7. Documentation.

8. Therapeutic milieu.

9. Special treatment procedures.

10. Emergencies.

    a. Code green.

    b. Code blue.

    c. Other codes used.

11. Infection control.

12. Fire safety code.

13. Physical management of aggressive behavior.

14. Orientation to the nursing unit(s).

These are but a few of the more important topics to be presented to the new nurse.

SUMMARY

When the student has completed Chapter 10, he/she should be able to:

- Assist with the preparation of a treatment plan.
- Assist with milieu therapy.

Review Questions

1. A patient who is scheduled for electroshock therapy is very concerned. The patient comes to you as a new staff member and asks "do people die from shock therapy?" Your most therapeutic response is:

    a. Only about 10% in the United States every year.
    b. You seem concerned about dying from the shock treatment, can you tell me why?
    c. You seem fearful of the scheduled treatment, can you tell me about your fears?
    d. Let us talk later, I have to give these medications right now.

2. The mental health staff members' ability to effectively communicate is most dependent on which of the following:

    a. Available resources to validate the content of the communication.
    b. The immediacy with which the staff attempts to interpret the communication.
    c. The staff's basic understanding of psychiatric terminology.
    d. How well the staff member listens and observes.

3. It is important for the staff to remember that the observed behavior has:
    a. Little to do with the patient's true feelings.
    b. Meaning.
    c. Purpose.
    d. Include b and c, and may represent the underlying feelings.

4. The main purpose for creating a treatment plan is to:
    a. Make sure there is compliance with the law.
    b. To establish a baseline of interventions to determine if the goals are realistic.
    c. To determine whether the treatment goals are going to provide adequate care.
    d. To organize care for the patient so that any staff member can contribute to the patient's care.

5. Which of the following is the primary reason for engaging the patient in group therapy?
    a. Gives the therapists a chance to supply information to the group.
    b. Provides for individual solutions to individual problems through discussion, discovery, and group actions on problems.
    c. Provides the mentally dull an opportunity to reason and form opinions through the group.
    d. Affords the therapist an opportunity to interact with several patients at one time, therefore, all the patients have equal professional counseling.

6. The primary focus of a group involved in recreation therapy is to:
    a. Provide diversional activities.
    b. Allow patients the opportunity to participate in physical (sports) activities.
    c. Give the patient time to be creative by doing fun activities that stimulate learning.
    d. Restructure life around games and pleasurable activities.

7. Reality therapy is best used in which of the following circumstances:
    a. Any time the patient is unable to tell you his/her name, the date, place, or purpose.
    b. During groups that are using reality therapy.
    c. Every time you meet a new patient.
    d. Only when ordered by the physician.

8. A locked patient unit is considered therapeutic because:
    a. The patients are confused and could harm themselves.
    b. There is less staff to work with the patients.
    c. The patients are acutely ill and require a safe, structured, and protective milieu.
    d. The patients are trying to behave themselves until they can get to the unlocked unit and escape.

9. Patients being treated on the adult psychiatric unit are there because:
    a. Its the only unit the court can commit them to.
    b. All of the patients have a psychiatric diagnosis.
    c. That is where their families want them.
    d. Psychiatric patients are sicker than other adult patients.

10. A patient's identity may be reinforced when he/she wears:

    a. His/her own street clothes.
    b. Hospital-provided attire.
    c. A loose-fitting uniform.
    d. Clothing that belongs to someone else.

CHAPTER 11

Psychotropic Medications

KEY CHAPTER OBJECTIVES

Upon completion of Chapter 11, the student should be able to identify satisfactorily correct answers to questions regarding the following knowledge areas:

- Identify psychotropic medications
- Identify the principles of medication administration
- Identify support groups
- Assist with medication administration

PSYCHOTROPIC MEDICATIONS

Psychotropic medications are those medications used in the treatment of the mentally ill. These medications are grouped by the psychiatric disorder that they are most likely to be used to treat.

- Antipsychotics
- Antidepressants
- Lithium
- Anxiolytics
- Stimulants
- Anticonvulsants

Let us review each of these groups by the following criteria: target symptom(s), generic name(s), trade name(s), and adverse (unwanted) effects. Not all trade names are listed in this writing.

Antipsychotics

A. The target symptoms of the antipsychotic group of medications are:

1. Agitation

2. Current (nonpersistent) delusions

3. Insomnia

4. Physical aggression (combative)

5. Loose associations (inability to process thoughts either continuously or sequentially).

6. Hallucinations

7. Paranoia

B. Although this is not an exhaustive listing, a representative sampling of antipsychotics, both by generic and trade name(s), includes:

GENERIC NAME	TRADE NAME
Chlorpromazine	Thorazine
✓ Clozapine	Clozaril
Fluphenazine	Prolixin
Haloperidol	Haldol ✓
Loxapin	Loxitane
Mesoridazine	Serentil
Perphenazine	Trilafon
Thioridazine	Mellaril
Thiothixene	Navane
Trifluoperazine	Stelazine

C. Potential adverse effects of the antipsychotics.

1. Cardiovascular effects

      a. Hypotension (low blood pressure).

      b. May be orthostatic if the patient is older.

      c. As the medication takes effect (1 to 2 weeks), hypotension may develop.

      d. If orthostatic hypotension should develop, patient should be taught to sit up for a few minutes before standing up.

      e. The antipsychotic medications that most frequently cause cardiovascular changes are Thorazine (chlorpromazine) and Mellaril (thioridazine).

2. Sedation

3. Photosensitivity

4. Weight gain

5. Extrapyramidal symptoms (EPS) associated with antipsychotics

      a. Dystonia—involuntary muscle movements that produce abnormal tensions and/or torsions (physical changes) in muscle configuration (shape), especially in the muscle groups of the face (eyes, tongue, etc.), neck, and upper back (torticollis).

      b. Parkinson—slow rigid movement

      c. Akathisia—restlessness

      d. Tardive—lip smacking

      e. Dyskinesia—distorted, involuntary muscle movements

6. The medications used for treatment of EPS or dystonic reaction includes:

TRADE NAME	GENERIC NAME
Cogentin	Benztropine
Benadryl	Diphenhydramine
Ativan	Lorazepam
Artane	Trihexyphenidyl

7. Pseudoparkinsonism may be manifested by one or more of the following objective signs:

      a. Drooling

      b. Pill rolling tremors of the fingers.

      c. Inability to maintain balance.

      d. Flat affect.

      e. Cogwheeling—periods of nonmotion followed by periods of motion of muscle groups.

      f. Bradykinesia—slow movement.

      g. Treated with same medications as dystonic reactions (*see* 6 above).

Antidepressants

A. Symptoms of depression that antidepressants may reverse.

1. Delusions
    a. Self-depreciation
    b. Guilt
    c. Hopelessness
    d. Somatic (body) focus
    e. Self-destruction or self-mutilating thoughts
2. Mood or feeling
    a. Sadness
    b. Pessimism
    c. Anger at self
    d. Irritability
3. Reduced physical and mental functioning
    a. Loss of appetite
    b. Inability to concentrate
    c. Unable to recall events (memory lapse)
    d. Fatigue
    e. Constipation
    f. Slowed or impaired thought process
    g. Diminished sex drive
4. Psychotic features
    a. Hallucinations
    b. Delusions that are very strong.

B. Medications (antidepressants) by generic and trade names. These medications may also be called tricyclics.

GENERIC NAME	TRADE NAME
Amitriptyline	Elavil
Amoxapine	Asendin
Desipramine	Norpramine
Doxepin	Sinequan
Imipramine	Trofranil
Nortriptyline	Pamelor
Trazodone	Desyrel✓
Fluoxetine	Prozac✓

The monoamine oxidase inhibitors (MAOI) are also used in the treatment of depression. These are listed by generic and trade names.

GENERIC NAME	TRADE NAME
Isocarboxizid	Marplan
Phenelzine sulfate	Nardil
Nialamide	Niamid
Tranylcyromine	Parnate

Special dietary restrictions apply for patients who are taking MAOIs. Special dietary considerations are foods or liquids that contain high concentrations of tryamine such as:

1. Cheese and dairy products that have been aged: cheddar, blue, brick, roquefort, sour cream, and yogurt.

2. Meats or fish that have been smoked, pickled, or fermented such as: beef or chicken livers, meats prepared with tenderizers, fermented sausages (pepperoni, salami, or summer sausage).

3. Alcoholic beverages such as: beer and ale, and red wines, especially Chianti.

4. Fruit and vegetables such as: overripe Avocado's, yeast extracts (marmite), bananas, figs (canned), raisins, soy sauce, bean curd.

Reactions of MAOIs with tryamine range from orthostatic hypertension to death.

C. Primary adverse effects of antidepressants:

1. Sedation

2. Cardiovascular effects

   a. Tachycardia

   b. Fainting

   c. Disrhythmias

   d. Myocardial infarction

3. Anticholinergic effects

   a. Dry mouth (xerostomia)

   b. Inability to sweat

   c. Urinary retention

   d. Constipation

   e. Psychosis

4. Weight gain

Lithium

A. Lithium is the treatment of choice for bipolar mood disorders, specifically, the manic phase.

B. When lithium is being administered, blood levels of lithium need to be monitored.

C. Lithium is a salt, such as lithium citrate, and may alter fluid levels in the body. Lithium is manufactured in a number of forms. (This list of lithium compounds is not all inclusive.)

1. Lithium citrate

2. Lithobid

3. Lithonate and Lithonate-S

4. Lithostat

5. Lithotabs

6. Carbolith

7. Eskalith

D. Adverse effects of lithium are:

1. Sedation (drowsiness)
2. Polyuria (excessive urine) and polydipsia (extreme hunger).
3. Weight gain
4. Muscle weakness and/or tremors

In addition to the adverse effects, there are toxic effects:

1. Nausea, vomiting, and diarrhea
2. Irregular and jerky tremors
3. Confusion and in some cases disorientation

Anxiolytics

Anxiolytics are sometimes referred to as minor tranquilizers. This group is called the benzodiazipines.

A. Anxiolytics target these symptoms
   1. Directly reduces the level of anxiety. The reduction of anxiety may facilitate the patient's ability to benefit from psychotherapy.
   2. Relieves the symptoms of withdrawal from substance abuse.
   3. Relieves the symptoms of delirium tremens.
   4. Relieves muscle tensions.
   5. Sometimes anxiolytics are used to potentiate the effects of narcotics, i.e., pre-operative medications.

B. Generic and trade names of anxiolytics in common use.

GENERIC NAME	TRADE NAME
Alprazolam	Xanax
Buspirone	Buspar
Chlordiazepoxide	Librium
Clonazepam	Klonopin
Diazepam	Valium
Flurazepam	Dalmane
Lorazepam	Ativan
Oxazepam	Serax
Temazepam	Restoril
Triazolam	Halcion

C. Most common adverse effects of anxiolytics:
   1. Sedation with higher doses
   2. Potential addiction
   3. Withdrawal, if the medication is stopped suddenly. Potential for seizures during withdrawal.
   4. Confusion

Stimulants

A. Stimulants are used for the following purposes:

    1. Energize the mind.

    2. Reverse the effect of depressant-type medications.

    3. Increase physical activity.

    4. Used illegally to produce a "high."

B. Generic and trade names of the stimulants:

GENERIC NAME	TRADE NAME
Amphetamine sulfate	Benzedrine
Dextroamphetamine	Dexedrine
Methamphetamine	Desoxyn
Pemoline	Cylert
Cocaine	—

C. Adverse effects of stimulants

    1. They are habituating and addictive substances with Schedule I recognition. Crack, a derivative of cocaine, is used illegally.

    2. Anorexia

    3. Insomnia

    4. Increases the blood pressure

    5. Causes tachycardia

    6. Patient may become highly agitated or irritable.

    7. Increases the possibility of seizures.

    8. May result in depression or psychosis.

    9. Caffeine is probably the most commonly used of the stimulant category.

Anticonvulsants

A. The category of medications that are used to control seizure activity.

B. Anticonvulsants by generic and trade names.

GENERIC NAME	TRADE NAME
Carbamazepine	Tegretol
Primidone	Mysoline
Phenobarbital sodium	Phenobarbital
Phenytoin	Dilantin
Valporic acid	Depakote

C. Major adverse effects of the anticonvulsants:

    1. Blood may not clot normally. Prolonged clotting time.

    2. Drowsiness.

3. Patient may not perform satisfactorily in the academic setting.

4. Patient may develop changes in skin, such as rash or thickening of epidermis, that can result in coarsening of facial features.

5. Nausea, vomiting, or diarrhea may occur.

6. Toxic effects may be nystagmus, ataxia, or seizures.

PRINCIPLES OF MEDICATION ADMINISTRATION

What follows is a general description of medication administration in a mental health facility; the basics are the same as in a general hospital. As you follow the policies and procedures you will recognize the differences.

As a licensed nurse, the LPN/LVN is the primary medication administration person. Therefore, it is important not only to follow these general guidelines but to be aware that certain hospitals will have their own specific policies and procedures.

A. The basics of medication administration.

1. Always wash your hands before you "pour" medications.

2. Always wash your hands after administering medications.

3. Always wash your hands when giving medications to patients—after direct patient contact.

B. The seven rights of medication administration.

1. Right patient—this must be verified before medications are to be given.

2. Right medication—this must be verified before medications are administered.

3. Right time—verified by the local policy and procedure.

4. Right route—verified from physician order and patient's physical condition to accept the medication via the ordered route.

5. Right dose—verified by physician order.

6. Right to refuse any medications they choose.

7. Right to request any medications that they feel they need.

C. When the physician orders the medication.

1. The order must contain medication name, route to be given, dose or strength, frequency of administration.

2. Medication orders can only be signed off by a licensed nurse (RN or LPN/LVN).

3. **Warning**: If the medication order is unclear, illegible, or does not contain any one of the required components, *call the physician*.

4. Doctors write orders generally on Physician's Orders Sheets. This means that the order needs to be transcribed onto the medication administration record.

5. Only a licensed nurse may accept telephone orders.

D. Transcribing the medication order.

1. Is always done as soon as possible (ASAP).

2. Is usually done in black pen.

3. Review *each* order.

4. Transcribe the order *exactly* as it appears.

5. Place a check next to each order (usually in front) as it is checked.

6. Annotate the date and time that the order was checked. Sometimes done in red pen.

7. Generally, the first initial and the full last name is written by the person checking the order. Included in the initialing will be the credential such as RN, LPN, or LVN.

E. The medication nurse's responsibilities.

1. Verify that the transcribed order has been transcribed correctly and accurately.

2. Review all medications to be given to the patient during the shift. This is done by checking each patient's medication administration record (MAR).

3. Before giving medications:

   a. Check start dates.

   b. Check discontinue dates.

   c. Check automatic stop dates.

   d. Check renewal dates—check local policy and procedure manual.

   e. Check for changes in medication orders.

   f. Check for new medication orders.

   g. Check for STAT or new doses.

   h. Check for PRN medications.

   i. Look for medication errors, transcription errors, or discrepancies.

   j. Be sure that the MAR has at least the following data:

      1) Patient name (stamped)

      2) Name of medication either generic or trade name is required.

      3) Correct ordered dose.

      4) Verify route of administration.

      5) The times that the medication is to be administered are correct.

      6) *Allergies.*

F. Pouring the medication

1. The medication cart and the medication room should both be locked when not in use.

2. Check the medication as you remove it from the medication cart or cabinet.

3. Check the medication against the verified Doctor Order as transcribed to the MAR. If there is *any* doubt about the Doctor Order—*call the Doctor!*

4. *Do not* open the medication (blister pack, etc) until you positively identify the patient.

5. Identify the patient.

    a. Ask the patient to tell you her/his name.

    b. Check the patient's ID band.

    c. Verify patient identity with a photograph.

    d. Ask another staff member to verify the patient's identity.

6. Open the medication package and administer the medication..

7. Stay with the patient and be certain that the patient swallows the medication.

8. *Never* give a medication unless you know what the medication's expected effects could be.

G. Recording the medications you have administered.

1. Enter name as appropriate including credentials on the MAR. This serves to identify the person who gave the medication.

2. Immediately after, *never before*, administration of the medication, write in the time given (using the correct date and shift column) and initial the entry.

3. If for any reason the medication was not given, follow the appropriate local policy and procedure.

4. *Never* leave the medication at the bedside and presume the patient has taken it.

H. After the medications have been given:

1. Observe the patient for any signs of adverse reactions or side effects. If the patient does experience an adverse reaction:

    a. Continue monitoring of the patient as appropriate.

    b. Notify the Team Leader at once.

    c. Document the extent of the adverse reaction and interventions in the Nurses Notes or Progress Notes.

    d. Complete any other required documentation as necessary.

2. Document any unusual occurrences or PRN's, STAT(s) doses, or reasons medications were *not* given or *not* taken by the patient, and to whom you reported the occurrences.

I. Other responsibilities.

1. If you have access to the narcotics cabinet, then you may be expected to count the narcotics at the beginning and the end of your shift.

2. *Never* give a medication that has been prepared by someone else!

3. Do teach patients about the medications that they are receiving.

4. Be sure to obtain and give any medications that are ordered STAT, NOW or ASAP.

5. Be sure that the appropriate consent forms have been properly signed before administering medications and other treatments as ordered by the physician.

Check local policy and procedure to determine what procedures and forms are needed.

6. Do not borrow medications from or between patients.

7. Medications are to be kept in individual patients containers and stored in drawers in the medication cart. Each patient's drawer is identified with name and room number.

8. *Never* attempt to change the label on a patient's medication. These should be given to the pharmacist.

9. Irritating and distasteful drugs should be diluted unless specifically ordered otherwise.

10. Cough syrups should not be diluted.

11. Acids and iron preparations should be given through a straw because they have a tendency to discolor the teeth.

12. Transdermal applications need to be completely removed with water/soap solution, and only be applied by the nurse wearing gloves.

13. Sublingual means under the tongue.

14. Record *only* the medications that you actually give.

15. Errors should be both reported and recorded.

PRACTICE MEDICATION EXAMINATION

In some instances, when applying for employment, you may be required to take and pass a Medication Administration test. This section of the book is to give you an idea of the kind of questions that you are likely to encounter. The examination may consist of one or more kinds of questions such as multiple choice, matching, true or false, fill in the blank, or other testing methods.

It is not so much the questions that appear here that are important, rather it is stimulating the mind to inquire into pharmacology of psychoactive medications. The key features to look for are the common routes of administration, optimal times for administration, usual doses, calculation(s) of the correct doses, effects and side effects, precautions such as narcotic class, pregnancy risk, interactions with other medications, and key teaching features associated with the medication.

All of the above information is in addition to the seven rights of medication administration.

Calculate the following:

1. Lithium citrate syrup 300 mg/ml. The order reads lithium citrate 450 mg, p.o. BID. The correct amount, in cc's is:

   a. 0.67 cc.
   b. 0.67 ml.
   c. 1.25 cc.
   d. 1.5 cc.

2. Dilantin suspension 125 mg/5 ml. The order reads give Dilantin 100 mg p.o., QID. The correct amount, in ml is:

   a. 1.25 ml.
   b. 1.67 ml.
   c. 2.25 ml.
   d. 4.00 ml.

3. Potassium chloride elixir 20 mEq/15 ml. The order reads: Give KCL elixir 30 mEq. p.o., A.C. and H.S. How many cc's will you give in one days time?

   a. 22.5 cc.
   b. 32.0 cc.
   c. 45 cc.
   d. 90 cc.

4. Mellaril concentrate 30 mg/ml. The order reads: give 0.1 g Mellaril p.o., TID. How many cc's will you give for one dose?

   a. 1.1 cc.
   b. 2.2 cc.
   c. 3.3 cc.
   d. 4.4 cc.

5. Thorazine concentrate 25 mg/cc. The order reads: give generic equivalent of Thorazine. Which of the following would you ask the pharmacist to deliver to you?

   a. Lorazepam.
   b. Chlordiazepoxide
   c. Thiothixene.
   d. Chlorpromazine.

6. Thorazine is classified as:

   a. An antipsychotic.
   b. An antianxiety (anxiolytic).
   c. An antidepressant.
   d. An anticonvulsant.

Match the correct Trade Name to the correct Generic Name.

7. Lorazepam	a. Tofranil
8. Amoxapine	b. Noctec
9. Amitriptyline	c. Ativan
10. Imipramine	d. Navane
11. Thioridazine	e. Elavil
12. Thiothixene	f. Librium
13. Chlopromazine	g. Mellaril
14. Chloral hydrate	h. Valium
15. Chlordiazepoxide	i. Asendin
16. Diazepam	j. Thorazine

Match the correct drug with correct dosage. The dosage numbers may be used more than once, if appropriate. One maintenance dose for the adult patient.

17. Halcion	a. 5 mg.
18. Dalmane	b. 1 mg.
19. Lanoxin	c. 0.5 mg.
20. Atropine	d. 50 mg.
21. Cogentin	e. 250 mg.
22. Lithium	f. 400 mcg.
23. Tylenol	g. 300 mg.
24. Benadryl	h. 30 mg.
25. Ampicillin	i. 325 mg.
26. Stelazine	j. 0.25 mg.

True or False questions. The entire question must be correct for the answer to be true. If any part of the question is false, then the answer is false.

_____ 27. Only a Registered Nurse may interpret and transcribe a medication order from the Doctor's order sheet to the medication administration record (MAR).

_____ 28. Mental health technicians may administer medications.

_____ 29. It is considered safe practice for a member of the nursing staff to administer medications prepared by another nurse.

_____ 30. If a patient questions a particular medication, he/she should be ignored and encouraged to take the medication in question.

_____ 31. Medications that are ordered before meals (AC), should be given about 30 minutes before each meal.

_____ 32. Different liquid medications must not be mixed together, unless ordered by the physician.

_____ 33. Patients taking tricyclic antidepressants are seldom suicidal, therefore. overdose is not a concern.

_____ 34. Lithium carbonate is recognized as the drug of choice for mania.

_____ 35. Lithium comes in oral and parenteral forms.

_____ 36. Lithium can be given in conjunction with a phenothiazine at the beginning of treatment, if necessary for a violent or agitated patient.

_____ 37. Any error in medication administration must be reported to the person in charge of the unit, but it is not necessary to complete any other forms.

_____ 38. It is not necessary to have a physician order, written, oral, or telephone, for every medication as you are assuming responsibility for the medication anyway.

_____ 39. Phenothiazines are potential photosensitizing agents.

_____ 40. A hypotensive crisis can result when a patient eats cheese or drinks wine while taking an MAO inhibitor.

_____ 41. Because tricyclic antidepressants lower the convulsion threshold, use with caution in patients with a history of seizures.

_____ 42. Mild drowsiness is commonly seen in the first days of therapy with benzodiazepines.

_____ 43. Thorazine concentrate does not have to be diluted before it is administered to a patient.

_____ 44. Extrapyramidal symptoms are reversible.

_____ 45. Extrapyramidal symptoms usually resemble a serious neurological disorder.

_____ 46. There have been misleading (false) reports of positive pregnancy tests on some patients that are receiving antipsychotic medications. These misleading tests are less likely to occur when a serum pregnancy test is ordered.

_____ 47. A consent form should be signed, *before* the medication Antabuse is administered.

_____ 48. Diazepam can be given to a patient who has acute narrow angle glaucoma.

_____ 49. Lorazepam is used to treat primary depressive disorder.

Write the symbols for each of the following:

50. drop   _____

51. one ounce   _____

52. one dram   _____

53. as necessary   _____

54. by mouth   _____

55. daily   _____

56. twice a day   _____

57. three times a day   _____

58. four times a day   _____

59. every six hours   _____

60. at bedtime   _____

61. before meals   _____

62. after meals   _____

63. one and one half grains _____

64. sufficient quantity   _____

65. immediately   _____

66. nothing by mouth   _____

67. right eye   _____

68. left eye   _____

69. both eyes   _____

In the space provided, give a primary use of each of the following medications.

70. Dilantin   _____

71. Adrenalin   _____

72. Lithium   _____

73. Sodium amytal   _____

74. Digitoxin   _____

75. Lasix   _____

76. Sodium bicarbonate   _____

77. Artane   _____

78. Dalmane   _____

79. Elavil   _____

80. Indocin   _____

81. Apomorphine   _____

Fill in the blanks based on the questions preceding the answer spaces.

What are the names of two commonly used drugs to relieve EPS?

82. _____

83. _____

List three side effects that you may encounter in a patient who is receiving phenothiazines:

84. _____

85. _____

86. _____

Name three signs or symptoms related to lithium toxicity.

87. _____

88. _____

89. _____

What are three critical steps that should be taken *before* the administration of Antabuse?

90. _____

91. _____

92. _____

Name four antidepressants (trade and generic names)

93. _____

94. _____

95. _____

96. _____

To prepare the patient for the blood test to measure her/his lithium level, you would teach the patient at least two essential items. They are:

97. _____

98. _____

List three signs of extrapyramidal symptoms.

99. _____

100. _____

101. _____

End of examination! Did you allow 101 minutes to complete the exam?

SUPPORT GROUPS

The names of these support groups are for the most part self-explanatory (this is a partial listing).

- Alzheimer's Support Groups
- Alcoholics Anonymous
- Rape Crisis
- Delta Society—for those mourning death of a pet
- Teen Courts and Teens Clubs—parenting and family dynamics
- Lupus Foundation
- Area Widowed Persons
- Council of Alcohol and Drug Abuse
- Jolly Janitors
- Palmer Drug Abuse Center
- Take Off Pounds Sensibly (TOPS)
- Women for Sobriety
- Fathers for Equal Rights, Wives and Grandparents Coalition
- AIDS Therapy group
- Epilepsy Foundation
- Family, Friends, and Caregivers—an AIDS support group
- Rational Recovery Systems—Nontraditional approach to drug abuse
- Depressive and Manic Depressive Association
- Female Victims of Physical Partner Abuse
- Toughlove Parent Support Group
- Overeaters Anonymous
- Recovery Inc
- Parents Anonymous
- Children's Separation and Divorce Support Group
- Phobia Society
- Impotents Anonymous
- Adult Children of Alcoholics

- Depression Support Group
- Care and Share Support Group—support for those dealing with life-threatening illness or bereavement
- Survivor's of Loved One's Suicides
- Cancer Conquerors
- Dysfunctional Families
- Sandwich Generation—those concerned about aging
- Dollars Anonymous—compulsive spenders
- Nicotine Anonymous
- Narcotics Anonymous
- Gender Alliance—for transgendered individuals and their families.

There are other resources. Many are available through the United Way in your area.

SUMMARY

As you review Chapter 11, keep in mind that one of the practical/vocational nurse's chief functions is to administer medications to the patients. You will be giving medications from this category: psychotropic medications.

You should not give any medication that you do not know the dose, route, frequency, or that does not have a written physician order. You should *positively* identify the patient that is to receive the medication before the medication administration. You should be familiar with the potential side and adverse effects of the medication as well as the toxic effects. You should have a medication source reference available to you that is current (no more than 3 years old).

1. A review of medications related to mental health.
2. A review of medication administration with emphasis on mental health.
3. Medication examination for review.

Why trust your cheesecake to anyone but PHILLY.

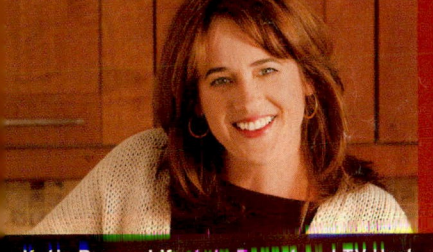

Katie Brown, Lifestyle Expert and TV Host.
KRAFT FOODS is a proud sponsor of the Katie Brown Workshop on Public Television.

PHILADELPHIA
New York Cheesecake

Prep: 15 min. plus refrigeration
Bake: 40 min.

6 HONEY MAID Honey Grahams, crushed
1 cup plus 3 Tbsp. sugar, divided
3 Tbsp. butter or margarine, melted
5 pkg. (8 oz. each) PHILADELPHIA
   Cream Cheese, softened
3 Tbsp. flour
1 Tbsp. vanilla
1 cup BREAKSTONE'S or KNUDSEN Sour Cream
4 eggs
1 can (21 oz.) cherry pie filling

During tests of plain NY style cheesecake made with PHILADELPHIA Cream Cheese versus store-brand versions, consumers rated PHILLY cheesecake better tasting.

HEAT oven to 325°F. Line 13x9-inch pan with foil. Mix crumbs, 3 Tbsp. sugar and butter; press onto bottom of pan. Bake 10 min.

BEAT cream cheese, sugar, flour and vanilla until blended. Add sour cream; blend. Add eggs, 1 at a time, mixing on low speed until blended.

BAKE 40 min. or until center is almost set. Cool completely. Refrigerate 4 hours. Use foil to lift cheesecake from pan.

TOP with pie filling and serve. Makes 16 servings.

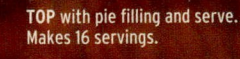

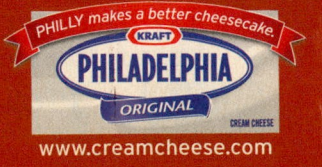

PHILLY makes a better cheesecake.
KRAFT
PHILADELPHIA
ORIGINAL
CREAM CHEESE
www.creamcheese.com

© 2008 Kraft Foods

Answers and Rationales to Review Questions and Practice Medication Examination

If you do not understand the answer, reread the content that pertains to that question. Be sure your answer agrees with the question. If the answer contains a threat, putdown, or judgment it is not an answer.

Chapter I

QUESTION	ANSWER	RATIONALE
1.	a.	Identification of self; we know ourself before we know others.
2.	b.	Rationalizing is the answer that completes the answer.
3.	b.	This is the definition of sublimation.
4.	b.	This is the definition of the Oedipus complex.
5.	b.	Answers a., c., and d. are inappropriate because these answers do not attempt to address the underlying feelings associated with hearing of voices. a. and c. are judgments made by the nurse and do not have any therapeutic value.
6.	a.	The ego is defined as the mediator between the superego and the id.
7.	c.	This is the definition of reaction formation.
8.	c.	This is the definition of displacement.
9.	a.	Retreating to an earlier time (regression) ensures a less threatening and more secure environment.
10.	c.	This is the definition of compensation.

Chapter II

1.	d.	The least threatening, most giving statement is also the most therapeutic one and the correct answer.
2.	d.	This is the best of the answers, as offering of self is the most therapeutic.

QUESTION	ANSWER	RATIONALE
3.	d.	Of the choices given, this is the best one as it is redirecting the thought process to a skilled listener. a., b., and c. are intrusive statements.
4.	b.	a., c., and d. contain untrue or negative statements. b. is the most therapeutic of these answers.
5.	a.	Until the patient can disclose feelings about death, he/she probably will be unable to deal with the feelings associated with the death of the relative. Remember, seek to find the underlying feelings that are causing the behavior.
6.	c.	Denial is a defense mechanism that reinforces behavior. Reality information is important, especially when delivered in a matter-of-fact style.
7.	b.	This is a suicide intervention. Is there a plan? If there is a plan, then you are dealing with an actively suicidal person.
8.	a.	Therapeutic communication is based on the disclosure of the greatest amount of information that can be gained from the patient. Yes and no questions and answers are restrictive, unless there is a follow-up open question.
9.	b.	The presence of another person is important to communication. Do not pressure the patient for an answer. The pressure may indicate to the patient you don't really care and that will certainly interfere with the communication process.
10.	d.	a. is untrue. b. is incorrect as nothing has been said about hostility. c. is true, but when you review d., it is the most correct of the four responses.

Chapter III

1.	a.	a. is correct because the patient is requesting to be admitted to the hospital for treatment. b., c., and d. are about circumstances which are a part of involuntary admissions.

QUESTION	ANSWER	RATIONALE
2.	b.	Involuntary admissions are a legal result of the lack or inability of the patient to recognize the need for mental health care.
3.	c.	APIE is the acronym for assessment, planning, intervention, and evaluation.
4.	c.	Objective means measurable. The only one of the answers that would result from a measurement is vital signs. Temperature, pulse, respiration, and blood pressure are measured by the nurse technician. The other answers are subjective, i.e., patient observations.
5.	b.	This is a feeling. Feelings are not measurable, therefore this is a subjective statement. The other responses are measurable and are objective.
6.	c.	a. is not measurable. b. is required by law, providing pills are ordered by the doctor. d. is not measurable and is too vague to have meaning. By elimination, c. is the correct answer.
7.	b.	A statement of evaluation or outcome is a measurable conclusion. a. is not correct as it is not measurable. b. is correct, "suicidal thoughts are gone." c. is not conclusive. d. is not measurable.
8.	b.	b. is correct as this answer comes directly from the definition of objective.
9.	d.	d. is the answer that most clearly answers the question. The other answers are subjective statements. a. is incorrect because it is only partially true given the d. answer. b. is totally irrelevant—does not have anything to do with the question. c. is objective data.
10.	a.	a. is correct. Assessment is the summation of objective and subjective data. The other answers are inappropriate in relation to this question.

Chapter IV

1.	c.	Least restrictive of these answers is c. verbal. a. and b. are mechanical or physical

QUESTION	ANSWER	RATIONALE
		restraints. d. is one of the highest forms of restriction after mechanical restraints.
2.	d.	Attempts to commit suicide are most likely to occur when the depression is lifting, therefore the correct answer is d. a. and b. are not likely compared with d. c. is not likely because when depressions are at their deepest point, there is general inability to move. Remember, you should always be alert for the presence of a suicide plan.
3.	c.	Why does the patient become depressed? a., b., and d. are helpful, but the real answer lies in (1) what caused the depression and (2) how to deal with those feelings.
4.	a.	The first step in dealing with any situation is assessment or what caused the crisis. Assessment means the collection of information (data). The other answers do not include information collecting.
5.	b.	Maintaining a line of sight and keeping the patient at no more than arms length at all times are the highest priority for the suicidal patient. The other answers are correct, but the highest priority is to prevent the death of the patient.
6.	a.	In the intervention of the aggressive patient a staff show of force will cause the patient to deescalate and regain self-control. b. is the next step and is implemented only if show of force is unsuccessful. c. medication is a possibility, but in itself will not alter the aggression for at least the length of time it takes for the medication to take effect, which is at least 20 minutes. d. would be used after verbal intervention.
7.	b.	b. is the correct answer as it is the answer that will identify suicidal thinking. a. is incorrect, you would not leave this patient alone. c. is incorrect because vital signs will not assess feelings. d. is not correct because the communication is not directed at thinking, specifically suicidal thinking.
8.	d.	Suicide precautions are ordered as described in d. a. is not correct because there is no

QUESTION	ANSWER	RATIONALE

guarantee that the patient will not commit suicide. b. is not correct because confining a suicidal patient to a quiet area will likely give the patient time to play out the plan and if possible, the attempt can be made. c. is not correct as it is given in the question that the patient is suicidal, that is, the patient has already stated to someone that he/she intends to commit suicide.

| 9. | d. | a., b. are distracters—answers given to distract from the content of the question. c. is true, but not as important to know as d. |
| 10. | b. | The real question here is which of the following is the least restrictive? Verbal inter ventions are always the preferred way to avert physical confrontation. |

Chapter V

1.	d.	Least likely is the one with the least amount of anxiousness (called anxiety) is depression. Think of these as opposites. a., b., and c. all involve a higher level of activity than depression. Depressed people are generally slow, withdrawn, and lethargic both physically and mentally.
2.	b.	Paranoids believe someone is out to get them. Suspicious is the giveaway in the answer. Suspiciousness does not appear in the other possible responses to the question.
3.	d.	a. and b. will not work because poverty is not a part of paranoia. c. is not correct because of the word poisoning. Grandiosity and persecution are the best answers.
4.	d.	This is the definition of psychosomatic diseases.
5.	d.	a. is not going to be possible because of the hyperactivity. b. is not correct because if the patient is eating, he/she is eating only small amounts of food at any one time. c. is inappropriate as this could be perceived as punitive and most likely is not possible because of the high level of activity.

QUESTION	ANSWER	RATIONALE
6.	c.	The question here is which of the following are characteristics of the border line personality. a. is not correct because the borderline person does not realize con sequences of her/his actions. b. is not cor- rect because they do not learn from any previous experiences. d. is not correct because these patients do not care and therefore, don't have to try to forget about the past.
7.	c.	a. is not correct as an attempt at keeping (interfering) with the ritual may only frus- trate the patient. b. is not correct as this would be "buying" into the behavior. d. is not correct as attempts to stop the behavior may create great anxiety and possibly accentuate the ritualistic behavior.
8.	a.	This is the definition of obsession or the thinking. Obsessions are recurring thoughts that are generally severe, frightening, and very unpleasant to the patient.
9.	c.	By definition, repetitive actions are termed compulsive behaviors. With compulsive behaviors there are strong underlying feel ings that should be dealt with such as mur- der and fear of infection.
10.	c.	It is the underlying feelings that need to be disclosed. a. is not correct because by focus ing on the amount of food consumed, counting calories, places emphasis on food—the one thing that an eating disorder patient absolutely does not want. b. is not correct as there is a high degree of self-con sciousness about food you would want to emphasize. d. is not correct because you do not know whether this patient is anorexic or bulimic.

Chapter VI

1.	a.	b., c., and d. simply do not fit the question.
2.	c.	a. is not true, actually psychotic responses are more severe than neurotic ones. b. is not correct because typically there will

QUESTION	ANSWER	RATIONALE
		be major reality gaps. d. is not correct because psychosis may be manifested in many ways—hallucinations are only one response.
3.	a.	Waxy flexibility is a symptom associated with catatonic type schizophrenia. b., c., and d. are all symptoms that may be associated with paranoid schizophrenia.
4.	b.	The four A's of schizophrenia and the only complete answer.
5.	d.	a., b., and c. are more associated with schizophrenics than with paranoids.
6.	a.	Projection is a mechanism to externalize feelings and known to us as hallucinations. b., c., and d. are defense mechanisms that are used by the mentally healthy unless they become pathologic with the user.
7.	b.	Yes and no answers limits and does not improve communication, therefore, by being the exception, b. is the correct answer.
8.	b.	b. answers the question the best in that there is acceptance of the unwillingness to enter into conversation, and there is understanding "I will sit here a while." a., c., and d. are inappropriate; acceptance is the more therapeutic intervention.
9.	d.	a. is inappropriate. b. is not appropriate. c. is appropriate, but the most appropriate answer is d.
10.	d.	Paranoid thinking is in progress with delusions of persecution. a. is not therapeutic. b. is buying into the delusional system—always avoid becoming a part of the system. c. is threatening to this patient because he/she is convinced that the events, as he/she describe them, are or have actually occurred.

Chapter VII

1.	d.	To recognize an alcoholic, a demonstrated dependency must exist, either psychological or physiological. If alcohol causes

QUESTION	ANSWER	RATIONALE
		an escape from a problem, then the dependency emerges and the underlying problem is not resolved. a., b., and c. are behaviors that are characteristic of an alcoholic.
2.	a.	The first hallucinations to appear will be visual after an acute intake episode. Delirium tremens is one time when visual hallucinations will be present.
3.	b.	Alcohol is a CNS depressant. Alcohol mixed with sedatives or other depressants may result in death.
4.	c.	Antabuse is the medication given to curtail alcohol consumption. If alcohol is consumed in the presence of Antabuse a violent physiological reaction will occur. Patients who have recently consumed alcohol (within the last 72 hours) should not be given Antabuse.
5.	b.	Confusion, fine muscular tremors and restlessness are the key features of delirium tremens.
6.	b.	The liver is the organ where the detoxification of alcohol occurs. Left untreated, the alcoholic's liver will begin to deteriorate, resulting in cirrhosis of the liver.
7.	a.	Alcoholics are generally unable to channel unacceptable behaviors into socially acceptable behaviors. The primary defense mechanism used by the addict is denial.
8.	b.	The physiologic reactions between alcohol and disulfiram are severe. The correct answer is b.
9.	b.	Drug seeking is the addict's way of bypassing or denying the addiction. Drug-seeking behavior is the mind set and the lifestyle. When addicts are admitted, medication is ordered to ease the withdrawal symptoms. The medications that help relieve the symptoms soon become the new drug of choice. Other substitute medications that alter thought processes are tobacco and caffeine.

QUESTION	ANSWER	RATIONALE
10.	b.	Some of each of a., c., and d. contain only one or none of the correct answer. Remember the entire answer must agree with the question.

Chapter VIII

1.	c.	a. is not correct as there is no mention of abuse in the question. b. would be correct if the talking is directed at the underlying cause. Because there is no indication of direction of the "talk," then this answer is not correct. d. is not possible until the feelings, the cause is identified, verbalized, and processed.
2.	c.	c. best describes the basis for token economics.
3.	d.	d. is the best answer of those given. a. is the result of anorexia nervosa. b. is incorrect. c. is the result of mind over body.
4.	a.	d. is not correct because only about 5% of bulimics are male. c. is not correct for the same reason as b. b. is true, but the better answer is a. Anorexia patients do not eat. Bulimic patients binge and then induce vomiting to lose weight.
5.	b.	a. is partially true. b. is the correct answer. c. is not correct because the pacts are rarely written. d. is not true.
6.	c.	If you did not correctly respond to this question, reread the material on mental retardation.
7.	a.	b. is not correct. c. is not correct. d. is not correct. The autistic's thoughts are not verbally expressed. When asked why autistics don't speak, the computer response from an autistic was "mouth locked."
8.	d.	The most important feelings to recognize during depression are hopelessness and helplessness. These feelings may lead to suicide. a. is not correct. b. is not correct. c. is an inappropriate response because anorexia is not a feeling, it is a disease.

QUESTION	ANSWER	RATIONALE
9.	d.	a. is not a direct cause of a rebellious or disturbed behavior. b. may cause a temporary disturbance, but it will soon pass. c. has nothing to do with behavior, actually 1 hour a day would be a control. d. is correct because if parents do not care or can not care because of need for employment then instability results. As the children grow they begin to establish their own rules, which may be immediately self-gratifying and self-serving. When the parent realizes what is occurring and attempt to enforce rules, the conflict begins. It is the initial indifference and/or rejection that triggers the eventual behavior.
10.	c.	The other answers are partially true but c. is correct. Everyone is responsible to report abuse of any kind.

Chapter IX

1.	c.	c. is the definition of defense mechanisms.
2.	b.	b. is the most therapeutic of the answers. a. is incorrect because a withdrawn patient should be encouraged to participate in activities. c. is not correct because we are not treating the withdrawnness of the family, but that of the patient. Shaming behavior is not effective when caring for the older patient. d. is not correct because this answer is too indirect and does engage the patient in an activity.
3.	d.	There are no two people that age at the same rate. Age is an individual event. b. and c. apply years to the aging process which is incorrect.
4.	b.	Unlike in the Eastern hemisphere, where the aging population is held in high esteem, in this hemisphere (western) the importance of the older population to society is perceived as having diminished importance.
5.	c.	The greatest liveliness is a diminished ability to hear. a. is not correct. b. is not correct

QUESTION	ANSWER	RATIONALE
6.	b.	because this answer has no foundation in the question. d. is not correct until an assessment is made of the acuity of hearing. Being therapeutic is the key to all nursing activities. To be therapeutic implies that there is sufficient knowledge and acceptance of the patient regardless of the condition or disease.
7.	d.	a. is an inappropriate response. Older patients will request more food if they are still hungry. b. is not totally correct in that only high fiber foods may be lacking in essential nutrients. The word *only* eliminates this answer. c. is not correct because, unless specifically ordered by the physician, liquified foods are not appropriate.
8.	c.	a. is not correct because confining a patient to a small area is inappropriate. b. is not correct because short would be better than long and aging patients are able to select their wearing apparel. d. is not correct because of the potential for burns associated with "open heaters." c. is the best answer.
9.	a.	Falls are the primary cause of injury of the older patient.
10.	d.	No one is certain about the cause of Alzheimer's disease.

Chapter X

1.	c.	c. is correct because it is a therapeutic response to identify the underlying feeling. a. is not correct. b. is not correct in that the patient has not said that he/she is fearful of death from shock treatment, but rather is seeking general information about EST. d. is not therapeutic.
2.	d.	d. is the best answer because it is the most complete answer. a., b., and c. are partial answers but are not complete answers.
3.	d.	a. is not correct because behavior is a direct result of feelings. b. and c. are correct and when included in d., form the best response.
4.	d.	The main purpose of the treatment plan is

QUESTION	ANSWER	RATIONALE
		to facilitate care of the patient in an organized fashion so all staff can participate. a. is a distractor to the question. b. is not completely correct in that a baseline is an assessment before the plan being designed. c. is not the best answer because the treat ment goals are established by the staff based on a completed assessment. d. is the best answer.
5.	b.	b. is the best answer. a. is partially true, but is not as complete as b. c. is a put-down by using the word "dull" and is not therapeutic. d. is incorrect in that the therapist is not the reason for the group, but rather the patient is the focus of group therapy.
6.	c.	c. is the best answer. a. is true but does not provide a primary focus for recreation ther apy. b. is true but misses the reason for the primary focus of RT. d. is not true because RT does not restructure life, rather it permits the patient to engage in activities that can reduce stress and foster social interactions.
7.	a.	a. is the best answer to this question. b. is true but is not the complete answer found in a. c. refers to assessment when a new patient is admitted. d. is not correct because a doctor's order is not required to use reality therapy by anyone.
8.	c.	c. is the most correct answer. a. is not correct because confusion is not a criteria for restricting movement. b. is not correct because generally there are more staff in a more restrictive milieu. d. is not correct.
9.	b.	a. is not true. b. is the best answer. c. is not true. d. is not necessarily true.
10.	a.	a. is the best answer of the one's available. b. is not correct because wearing hospital clothes may be disastrous to the men tal health patient in that it deidentifies the patient. c. is not correct for the same reason. d. is not correct because it is inappropriate.

QUESTION	ANSWER	RATIONALE

Chapter XI

1.	d.	d. is the correct calculation. If 1 ml has 300 mg of lithium citrate, then how many cc's will have 450 mg of lithium? a. 0.67 x 300 = 201 mg wrong dose. b. same as a. c. 1.25 x 300 = 375 mg, which is a wrong dose. d. 1.5 x 300 = 450 mg, correct dose.
2.	d.	125 mg/5 ml. How many ml = a dose of 100 mg? By dividing 125 by 5 we know that each ml has 25 mg of medicine. a. 1.25 ml x 25 = 31.25 mg, a wrong dose. b. 1.67 ml x 25 = 41.75 mg, a wrong dose. c. 2.25 ml x 25 = 56.25 mg, a wrong dose. d. 4 ml x 25 = 100 mg, the correct answer.
3.	d.	20 mEq/15 ml = 30 mEq/X; X = 22.5 cc for one dose. You are supposed to give four doses, one before each meal and one at bed time—a total of four doses. If one dose is 22.5 cc, then multiply by 4 to find the total cc's given in 1 day is 90 cc. Be sure you read the questions very carefully and as importantly read every answer.
4.	c.	Divide 100 mg by 30 mg = 3.3 cc.
5.	d.	The generic equivalent of Thorazine is chlorpromazine.
6.	a.	Thorazine is a major antipsychotic.
7.	c.	
8.	i.	
9.	e.	
10.	a.	
11.	g.	
12.	d.	
13.	j.	
14.	b.	
15.	f.	
16.	h.	
17.	c.	
18.	h.	
19.	j.	
20.	f.	
21.	b.	
22.	g.	

QUESTION	ANSWER
23.	i.
24.	d.
25.	e.
26.	a.
27.	F
28.	F
29.	F
30.	F
31.	T
32.	T
33.	F
34.	T
35.	F
36.	F
37.	F
38.	F
39.	T
40.	T
41.	T
42.	T
43.	T
44.	T
45.	T
46.	T
47.	T
48.	F
49.	F
50.	gtt.
51.	oz.
52.	dr.
53.	PRN
54.	p.o.
55.	q.d.
56.	BID
57.	TID
58.	QID
59.	q6h
60.	at HS
61.	AC
62.	PC
63.	gr. 1 1/2
64.	qs
65.	STAT
66.	NPO

QUESTION	ANSWER	
67.	OD	
68.	OS	
69.	OU	
70.	Anticonvulsant.	
71.	Cardiac stimulant.	
72.	Antimanic.	
73.	Sedative hypnotic.	
74.	Cardiotonic.	
75.	Diuretic.	
76.	Alkaline agent.	
77.	Antiparkinson's.	
78.	Sedative hypnotic.	
79.	Antidepressant—tricyclic.	
80.	Nonsteroidal antiinflammatory.	
81.	Emetic.	
82.	Cogentin.	
83.	Benadryl.	
84.	Sedation.	
85.	EPS	
86.	Hypotension.	
87.	Polyuria.	
88.	Weight gain.	
89.	Muscular weakness.	
90.	The patient must agree to take the medication.	
91.	Do Not give to the patient if alcohol has been consumed within the last 72 hours.	
92.	The patient must be taught not to use external alcohol such as after shave etc.	
93.	Amitriptyline	Elavil
94.	Desipramine	Norpramine
95.	Imipramine	Trofranil
96.	Trazadone	Desyrel
97.	The blood level of lithium has to be measured.	
98.	Encourage fluid intake.	
99.	Dystonia.	
100.	Tardive dyskinesia.	
101.	Parkinson's movements	

INDEX